ALKALINE DIET

The Revolution of Eating Habits to stay Healthy and Find the Best Shape. A complete Program to Regain a Healthy Balance of the Body with Alkaline Foods and lose Weight Quickly.

KELI BAY

CONTENTS

INTRODUCTION

WHAT IS THE ALKALINE DIET?

The alkaline diet, or the alkaline ash diet, takes a whole new approach to what we consume. It does not consider the proportions or the nutritional composition of foods like other diets do. Instead, it considers the effects the different types of metabolic waste produce after food has been digested and assimilated. The type of food determines the nature of its metabolic waste. Therefore, food containing acid compounds or acidic elements produces acidic waste, whereas alkaline foods produce alkaline metabolic waste. The experts who first suggested the idea of an alkaline diet for a healthier living say that acidic metabolic waste is harmful to bodily health as it can disrupt the optimal pH levels within the body which are essential to regulating enzyme function, hormone production, and other metabolic reactions. That is why the alkaline diet was proposed, it can help maintain the internal alkaline environment through the production of alkaline metabolic waste.

WHAT IS PH?

Put simply, a pH value defines the measure of alkalinity, or basicity and acidity, of a substance or an environment. There is an optimal pH value required to carry out basic metabolic functions. On the scale of 0-14, substances with 0-6 pH values are considered acidic, those having 7 are neutral, and ones with 8-14 pH values are basic in nature. Human blood is also slightly alkaline, having a value of 7.35-7.45 on the pH scale. This pH value is optimal for all the components carried by the blood in the body. Since blood is pivotal to all metabolic functions in the body, it carries hormones, enzymes, nutrients, and other essential substances, it's important to maintain the necessary pH level.

HOW DOES FOOD AFFECT YOUR BODY?

Optimal pH is vital to support normal metabolic functions. When we eat substances that can produce acidic by-products or end products, they will likely end up in our blood and may lower its pH value, making it more acidic. Once that balance is disrupted, all the functions associated with the blood and the components present in it are also slowed down or they are not properly executed in the body. Moreover, acidic foods can also be harmful to the microbes residing in the human intestine as they require a high pH level to survive. Contrarily, if we eat foods that can support a normal pH level in the body, whether in the blood or in the cells, it can be very healthy for us.

HOW DOES THE ALKALINE DIET HELP?

The principle on which the alkaline diet works is simple: do not eat foods that are considered acid-forming or acidic. It means that substances that have a tendency to produce acidic metabolic waste or by-products should be avoided to maintain natural pH levels in the body. Even when it comes to digestion, it is only the stomach that digests food in an acidic environment; the same food has to be transformed into an alkaline state before reaching the intestines to complete digestion and assimilation. The alkaline diet, therefore, recommends consuming foods which produce alkaline metabolic waste or end products.

PROOF THAT THE ALKALINE DIET IS USEFUL

A 2010 cancer study suggests that acidic food can hinder the successful treatment of cancer while depriving the body of its optimal metabolic conditions (Diet and cancer prevention: Contributions from the European Perspective Investigation into Cancer and Nutrition (EPIC) study—Carlos A. Gonzalez, 2010). Experts discovered that when cancer patients were given alternative alkaline diets, they became healthier and more resilient against the disease. Similarly, there is evidence from a 2017 study that tells us about the harm an acidic diet can have and how it can negatively affect kidney health (Reducing the Dietary Acid Load: How a More Alkaline Diet Benefits Patients with Chronic Kidney Disease- Carolina Passey, 2017). In contrast to this, the alkaline diet has not only proven to be effective in preventing kidney problems, but it is also good for heart health, regulation of hormones, and boosting brain function.

THE MICROBIOME AND ITS ROLE IN ALKALINITY

The microbiome is a whole community of microbes that live inside the human digestive system. We are familiar with the fact that there are numerous nutrients that cannot be digested by human-produced enzymes. These microbes present in the gut help us digest those nutrients and break them down into simpler components. They can survive only in an alkaline environment and, therefore, they also produce alkaline by-products to maintain the pH around them. That is why they are both contributors to and beneficiaries of this alkalinity. Also, when we eat acid-forming food, it is likely to disturb this naturally occurring microbiome.

THE RATIO OF MACROS AND HOW THAT AFFECTS ALKALINITY

Every macronutrient has a different composition; some carry more acidic components than others. Proteins, for example, have amino acids as their monomers (the basic molecular structure which makes up a protein chain.) These are acidic in nature and overconsumption of complex proteins like those present in red meat can likely affect the alkalinity level in the body. Less complex amino acids, on the other hand, are not completely restricted. It is more about the proportion of protein intake. Carbohydrates usually contain fewer acids. However, foods containing carbohydrates are considered acid-forming. Fats have fatty acids which can also negatively affect alkalinity, especially animal fats which are restricted on the alkaline diet.

HEALTH CONDITIONS IMPROVED BY ALKALINE DIET

The following are the health conditions and problems in which the alkaline diet can complement medical treatment and therapies:

- Diabetes
- Muscle Pain
- Gout
- Arthritis
- Bloating
- Cancer
- Insomnia

ALKALINE WATER

Pure water is neutral, and it has a pH value of 7. Alkaline water, on the other hand, has a higher value of 8 to 9 on the pH scale. This water can be consumed to help maintain the alkalinity within the human body, especially the gut and blood. It is used for various purposes, from detoxification to countering the effects of aging, reducing obesity, and fighting cancer.

ALKALINE DIET FREQUENTLY ASKED QUESTIONS

- What is the difference between alkaline food and the Acid Reflux diet?

The acid reflux diet is mainly concerned with the role of the stomach and its proper functioning. This diet was created to reduce the acidity in the stomach and stop the overproduction of hydrochloric acid (HCl) in the stomach. However, the alkaline diet is focused on the pH balance within the body, whether it is in the gut, blood, or other organs.

- How can alkaline food control obesity?

The alkaline diet recommends a reduction in intake of complex carbs, sugars, and saturated fats. All these food items are mainly responsible for obesity.

- Does cooking change the alkalinity of food?

No, this is far from reality. The acidic and basic character of the food is its chemical property, it does not change during overheating or cooking.

ALKALINE AND ACID-FORMING FOODS

The food we eat can be categorized into two main groups with respect to the alkaline diet. The one which has the tendency to produce acidic metabolic waste is known as acid-forming, whereas the food which can produce alkaline metabolic products after digestion is known as an alkaline-forming food. Let's take a look and categorize different ingredients on the basis of this property.

ACID-FORMING FOODS

- Coffee and other caffeinated drinks
- Beef, pork, lamb, fish, and chicken
- Popcorn
- Cornmeal, rye
- Rice: white, brown, or basmati
- Wheat germ
- Colas
- Cheese
- Pasta
- Alcoholic drinks
- Soy sauce
- Ketchup
- Sweetened yogurt
- Mustard
- Refined table salt
- Mayonnaise
- Tobacco
- White vinegar
- Nutmeg

ALKALINIZING FOODS

- Peas
- All vegetable juices
- Most herbal teas
- Beans: string, soy, lima, green, and snap
- Arrowroot flour
- Sprouted seeds of alfalfa, radish, and chia
- Grains: flax, millet, quinoa, and amaranth
- Potatoes
- Nuts: fresh coconut, almonds, pignolia, and chestnuts

- Unsprouted sesame
- Fresh unsalted butter
- Whey
- Plain yogurt
- Fruit juices
- Garlic
- Cayenne pepper
- Gelatin
- Most herbs
- Miso
- Most vegetables
- Unprocessed sea salt
- Most spices
- Vanilla extract
- Sweeteners: raw, unpasteurized honey, dried sugar cane juice (Sucanat), brown rice syrup
- Brewer's yeast

AVOID ACIDOSIS

THE RIGHT BODY PH

Let's begin with a little refresher in chemistry class and remind ourselves about what pH is. A simple definition is how much hydrogen ion concentration there is in our body. The initials pH is short of "power of hydrogen". The "p" stands for "potent" or the German word for power and "H" stands for the element symbol for hydrogen. The pH scale ranges from one to 14. Seven is neutral. A pH of less than seven will be acidic. Solutions that have a pH of more than seven are alkaline.

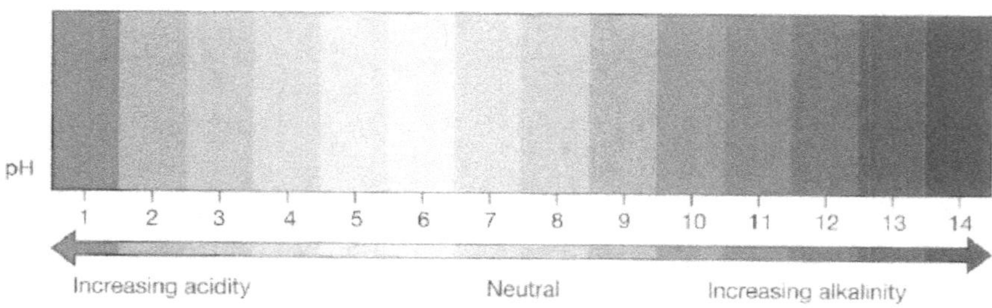

In order for us to have good health, our bodies need to be a little bit alkaline. Our blood's pH and other cellular fluids should be around a pH of 7.365 to 7.45. It is important to realize that pH levels will vary a lot throughout the body. Some parts will be acidic while others will be alkaline. Basically, there isn't a set level. Our stomachs are loaded with hydrochloric acid and this gives it a pH of between 2 to 3.5. This makes it very acidic. It needs to be this acidic so it can break down the foods that we consume and kills harmful bacteria. Our saliva ranges from pH levels of 6.8 to 7.3. The skin has a pH level of 4 to 6.5. This acts as a protective barrier from the environment. Our urine has a pH that will vary from alkaline to acid. It all depends on what your body needs in order to balance our internal environment due to the foods we eat.

ACIDS AND DIGESTION

The measurement that is most important will be your blood's pH. It needs to keep in a very narrow range between 7.365 and 7.45. This might seem simple but instead of our pH operating within a mathematical scale, it operates within a logarithmic scale in multiples of ten. This means that it will take ten times the amount of alkalinity to be able to neutralize an acid. If there is a jump from six to seven, it might not seem like much but it will take ten times the amount of alkalinity to neutralize this amount. Basically, a pH of five will be 100 times more acidic than a pH of seven. A pH of four will be 1,000 times more acidic. Does this help you understand?

Don't begin stressing about staying in or falling out of that range. Remember your body is pretty great at regulating the pH of your blood. Your body doesn't "find" the balance. It has many parts that do this and keeps the blood's pH between 7.365 and 7.45 at all times. If you make a poor lifestyle and diet choices, your body works harder to keep the balance. If you want to address the inflammation and acidity in your body by changing your dietary choices to foods that are more alkaline, it will help balance your system and bring your body back to its best vitality.

Even the smallest of alterations to the pH level of different organisms can cause massive problems. Because of environmental concerns like increasing the deposition of CO_2 in the ocean, its pH level has dropped from 8.2 to 8.1 and the many different life forms that live in the ocean have suffered a lot. The pH level is critical for plant growth and it can affect the mineral content of foods we consume. The human body, soil, and minerals in the ocean are buffers that help maintain the optimal pH level. When there is a rise in acidity, minerals decrease.

WHEN THE BODY RISKS BECOMING ACIDIFIED

You should know how important it is to maintain a balanced pH. This portion will tell you about the fatal consequences of changes to the pH. If the pH level in the body gets too alkaline, a symptom called Alkalosis is going to happen. When the body is put under these conditions, you will begin to experience a loss of electrolytes, liver disease, lower oxygen levels, etc.

Here are some symptoms of alkalosis:

- Tingling in the face
- Problems breathing
- Seizure
- Sudden onset of muscle spasms
- Twitching
- Light-headedness
- Confusion

On the other hand, if the body starts to get too acidic, your body will enter into a state of acidosis. There are some risks to acidosis like:

- Lethargy
- Breathlessness
- Fatigue
- Confusion
- Kidney damage
- Insulin resistance
- Diabetes

- Increased risk of heart disease
- Renal complications
- Lactic imbalance
- Respiratory problems
- Metabolic problems

Acidosis can be brought on by a diet that isn't balanced and that contains a lot of animal products with only a few vegetables and fruits. Here are some symptoms of acidosis:

- Vomiting
- Nausea
- Increased heart rate
- Arrhythmia
- Diarrhea
- Muscle weakness
- Seizures
- Coughing
- Shortness of breath
- Confusion
- Sleepiness
- Headache
- Loss of consciousness
- Coma

THE BENEFICIAL EFFECTS OF THE ALKALINE DIET

Here is a rundown of all the advantages the alkaline diet offers your body:

- It can increase your sex drive and enhances sexual power.
- It can slow down the natural aging process and will keep you looking fresher and younger.
- It can improve the health of your teeth and gums.

- The alkaline diet can increase your body's available energy and will keep it energized throughout the day.
- It will help you lose weight.
- It can help improve your body's immunity and can protect you from developing cancer.
- It can help boost how the body absorbs vitamins and minimizes the deficiency of magnesium.
- It can help lower chronic pain and inflammation.
- It will lower the risk of stroke and hypertension.
- It can help protect bone mass and muscle density.

STRATEGIES FOR ELIMINATING TOXINS AND OVERWEIGHT

When you decide to get healthy, you can't expect to be perfect on the first day and you can't deprive yourself of foods that you really enjoy. To have success when learning to eat alkaline and keeping this lifestyle, you need to learn moderation since life is about balance. Deprivation is the reason behind the failures of most diets. Finding the perfect balance can be confusing and challenging when you first begin this new lifestyle. In order to get the most benefits out of the alkaline diet is to use the 80/20 rule. This means that in order to keep a healthy internal environment, you need to try to eat a diet that contains around 80 percent alkaline-forming foods and the remaining 20 percent coming from acid-forming foods. Basically, refined starches and animal proteins are acid, whereas, fruits, vegetables, and beans are alkaline.

It is easy to put this into play if you just visualize your plate and think about food groups. To have optimal health, you need to eat plant proteins, healthy fats, tubers, vegetables, and fruits that take up 80 percent of your plate. Other acidic foods and starches will take the remaining 20 percent. If you can do this for every meal, this will guarantee your diet will always be 80 percent alkaline and 20 percent acid. You might be tempted to get rid of all alkaline foods from your diet. This would be a huge mistake. High protein foods like beans, fish, milk, and meat are acidifying but your body has to have protein so it can repair and rebuild your body.

If you like tofu that is mildly alkaline and low acid then go ahead and put it into your diet. Just eat it in moderation. Even though it isn't a high protein food, you can even have a piece of chocolate or a slice of birthday cake now and then. The keywords are moderation, balance, and shifting your diet from constantly eating acid-forming foods to a diet where they begin taking up a small part of your plate. Slowly bring back in foods that have the most impact and before you realize what is happening, all that good will outweigh the bad and your energy and health will increase.

THE RIGHT FOODS

Eating alkaline means you will be consuming plenty of fruits and vegetables, but it doesn't mean you will be eliminating everything on the acidic spectrum, which includes (surprise!) certain whole grains and legumes that can be highly beneficial to your health and well-being.

This will provide insight into which foods are the best options and which foods you should generally limit or avoid; it's essentially a shopping list for the utmost success. We also debunk some current myths about the alkaline diet. This part prepares you for the next stage of your journey, including getting your pantry ready, shopping for ingredients, and planning your first month of the alkaline diet using a carefully devised meal plan for optimal nutrition.

FOODS TO EAT

For the most part, fruits and vegetables are considered alkaline, while meat, dairy, and highly processed foods are viewed to be more acid-forming.

The concern among supporters of the acid-ash hypothesis is that high levels of acid ash in the body overtax the body's acid-base regulatory mechanisms, which disrupts other regulatory functions in the body. That being said, there remains no scientific validity supporting the notion that you can actually affect your blood pH through consuming alkaline-rich foods. Furthermore, your body may be more capable of regulating blood pH than you think.

We may not entirely understand the etiology in which highly inflammatory conditions, such as kidney disease, develop, and progress. But as we learned, implementing a diet rich in plant foods and limited in animal proteins, dairy, and unprocessed foods can shape a healthier outlook for a relatively healthy individual. Alkaline foods are good for your health, primarily because they are plant foods. Plant foods contain a wide variety of essential vitamins, minerals, amino acids, and antioxidants. In their whole form, they provide a synergy of nutritional benefits. Let's take a look at some.

- Dark Leafy Greens

Dark leafy greens include kale, spinach, chard, arugula, and green-leaf and romaine lettuce. They deliver an array of nutrients including vitamins A, C, and K, folate, fiber, magnesium, calcium, iron, and potassium.

- Non-Starchy Vegetables

Non-starchy vegetables include radishes, mushrooms, artichokes, asparagus, broccoli, cauliflower, cucumber, carrots, jicama, peppers, and, of course, leafy greens. They come in a variety of colors and textures, and like leafy greens, they provide very few calories per gram of weight.

- Fruits

When we consider fruits, we are looking at plant foods that not only provide a naturally sweeter taste but also contain a variety of antioxidant nutrients and essential vitamins and minerals. Fruits are delicious on their own, paired with nuts or nut butter, in salads and healthy green smoothies, and even added as natural sweeteners to balance out flavors in bitter greens like arugula and some savory dishes like curries.

• Nuts

Although nuts are high in calories, they offer healthy monounsaturated and polyunsaturated fatty acids such as omega-3s that are essential for brain function and hormonal regulation in the body. So, include these in your diet, but exercise portion control—1 ounce (2 tablespoons) is considered one serving. Nuts provide nutrients such as magnesium (which helps regulate blood pressure) and immune-supportive vitamin E. According to research, nuts may help lower bad cholesterol, lower levels of inflammation related to heart disease, and improve the structure and lining of your arteries. The American Heart Association suggests consuming 1.5 ounces (3 tablespoons) of unsalted nuts per day, four times per week.

• Seeds

Like nuts, seeds are also calorie-dense but full of nutrients. They also provide polyunsaturated and monounsaturated fats, as well as fiber and nutrients like vitamin E. Consumed in small portions, they can be part of a healthy diet. Like nuts, seeds may help regulate blood sugar (as they are low in carbohydrates and include dietary fiber) and blood pressure. Top your salads or soups with a light sprinkling of seeds to provide a delicate crunch, a bit of flavor, and some added nutrients to your plate.

• Olive Oil and Avocado Oil

These oils are included in your healthy fats because they can help provide you with the essential fatty acids you need. The monounsaturated and polyunsaturated fats in these healthy oils benefit the brain, nerves, skin, nails, and hormonal regulation, too! Used sparingly to lightly coat leafy greens (and when used in combination with spices and other foods), they help carry and distribute flavor to your palate.

- Beans and Other Legumes

These plant foods are special because they are not only rich in complex carbohydrates, but also good sources of protein, making them a part of two food groups. Additionally, they are rich sources of fiber and essential B vitamins.

- Whole Grains

Intact whole grains such as quinoa, buckwheat, and brown rice provide some protein, as well as the benefit of complex carbohydrates, and their fiber contents ultimately assist in blood sugar control. They bring B vitamins to the table, as well as a variety of other heart-healthy nutrients, including iron, magnesium, and phosphorus.

- Tofu and Soybeans

Soybeans (known as edamame in their whole, cooked form) can be processed into tofu, which, like its base component, is a good protein source. Yes, tofu is processed, but not highly processed, and thus it doesn't contain a lot of additives. Generally, it is made up of three ingredients: soybeans, water, and a coagulant. Tofu offers the benefit of a convenient source of protein that can easily translate into many different dishes due to the variety of textures available and its mild flavor.

- Apple Cider Vinegar

This vinegar is highly touted in many popularized versions of the alkaline diet. The benefit of this tangy acid (which, like lemon, leaves an alkaline ash in the body) is that its flavor is so intense, just a little can add a lot of flavor to your food. As a fermented food, it may help support digestive health.

FOODS TO AVOID

Although this diet is not highly restrictive, there is a very good reason to limit or avoid certain foods. Many of the following foods are not only more acidic, they are also more inflammatory, especially if consumed in large amounts. Even though some of the foods on this list provide some nutritional benefit (e.g., meat is a protein-rich food that contains the essential vitamin $B^{12)}$, it is best to focus more on your fruits, veggies, intact whole grains, beans, and legumes. Below are some reasons, beyond their acidity, to limit or avoid the following foods.

- Red Meat

Red meat contains phosphorus, an essential nutrient you can also obtain from plant foods. It is also a very good source of protein and vitamin B^{12}. However, it is higher in saturated fat than other proteins, such as chicken, fish, and vegetable proteins. Saturated fats have been correlated with cardiovascular disease risk factors. There is strong evidence that consuming red meat and processed meats causes cancer, particularly colorectal cancer, according to the American Institute for Cancer Research, and a large body of scientific evidence links the high intake of red meat and processed meats to greater risks of heart disease, cancer, and diabetes, according to Harvard Health.

- Processed Meats

Processed meats include sausages, ham, corned beef, smoked meats, and dried meats, which are preserved through curing, salting, smoking, or drying. High intake of processed meats has been implicated in chronic disease, including high blood pressure, cancer, and heart disease.

- Added Sugars

Added sugars include, but are not limited to, refined white sugar, brown sugar, corn syrup, rice syrup, dextrose, honey, malt sugar, and molasses—many of which are found in highly processed foods. Diets high in added sugars are widely known to promote insulin resistance and weight gain. Scientific evidence also reveals that high sugar intake can increase cardiovascular risk, including raising triglycerides and LDL ("bad") cholesterol and promoting inflammation, blood platelet disruption, and oxidative stress that contributes to atherosclerosis (hardening of the arteries).

- Dairy

Dairy includes milk, yogurt, kefir, butter, and any of those foods processed from the milk of an animal (e.g., cow and goat milk). Many dairy foods have the benefit of containing calcium and protein, and some, such as yogurt and kefir, contain probiotics. Dairy can contribute to allergies or sensitivities in certain individuals, and some science supports that it can be inflammatory in the body (although there is conflicting evidence on this matter). Regardless, limiting dairy is not detrimental, as you can get plenty of calcium and protein from a wide variety of plant foods.

- Highly Processed Grains

Highly processed grains include bread, muffins, crackers, tortillas, cakes, and pastries. The processing of wheat, rice, and other whole grains into flour (an ingredient in these foods) removes the outer fiber-rich layer and nutrient-dense germ, leaving behind the starch, which is rapidly converted to sugar in the body—a process that can adversely affect blood. Furthermore, highly processed foods contain additives, including sugars, sodium, chemicals, stabilizers, and more, that have little benefit for the body, and some of these (like BHT added as a preservative) are considered toxic. Additionally, some unexpired, highly processed foods may contain trans fats if they were manufactured before 2018 when the fats were banned.

- Alcohol

Wine, beer, vodka, and gin are broad examples of alcohol people may enjoy. Studies implicate excessive alcohol intake with blood pressure and heart disease risk. Furthermore, many alcoholic drinks include added sugars or syrups—further increasing the sugar content of the drink.

- Coffee

Caffeine may be beneficial for its immediate energy boost, but these effects don't last long. Studies that support its health contributions (as well as deficits to optimal health) are conflicting. Dependency on caffeine can reduce the intake of nutrient-dense options if you use it constantly to boost your energy to get through the day.

- Chocolate

When we refer to chocolate, we are generally not talking about the cocoa bean itself, but rather the product it gets processed into, whether it's chocolate chips, a chocolate bar, or cocoa powder for hot cocoa. Consuming sugar-free chocolate is not much better; many people feel that artificial sweeteners permit you to consume more artificially flavored foods with less nutritional value. Not only does the chocolate we eat contain added sugars or sugar substitutes, but it's also calorie-dense and contains caffeine.

- Soda

Sodas are often processed with added sugars or sugar substitutes (non-nutritive sweeteners). Sugar substitutes are highly processed and may not have the overall health benefits one might expect, despite containing little to no calories or sugars. Furthermore, sodas don't provide much nutritional value beyond the phosphorus they contain (which actually may be excessive for anyone who overconsumes soda). Additionally, soda is a diuretic and thus dehydrating. Drinking soda to quench thirst is actually counterproductive, as it often replaces necessary recommended water intake.

- Protein Supplements

Protein supplements include blends of vegetable proteins such as pea protein or animal-derived proteins such as whey protein or collagen. It is important to note that many of these powders or blends are highly processed. Although some supplements may contain a convenient source of protein (and perhaps other additional nutrients), they are highly processed and thus exposed to chemicals used in the processing. It is better to get your nutrients from whole foods.

THE PRACTICAL RULES

A meal prep guideline is there to help you organize your life in a way that will ensure you always eat healthy meals without having to spend a lot of time preparing them.

MEAL PLANNING

Generally speaking, meal planning makes your life easier especially if you're on a diet that requires sticking to a specific eating plan. In the case of the Alkaline diet, there is a list of foods that are allowed and those that are not. This actually makes your meal prepping very easy because there is a limited list of foods so all you have to do is shop according to this list. Besides, this diet is practically vegan, the focus is on fruits and vegetables so meal prepping revolves around soups, salads, smoothies, juices, and steamed vegetables. Although this may not be always possible, it's best to use foods that are in season.

The basics of meal prepping are meal planning which starts with selecting the recipes, deciding how many meals you are going to prepare (e.g. three meals per day or just one, the main one), and for how many days you want to plan ahead. Although planning is only the first step, it is the most important one.

SHOPPING FOR INGREDIENTS

Once you have an idea of what meals you are going to prepare and for how many days, you should make a shopping list. If you are prepping a meals for several other people besides yourself, you may have to consider their preferences. This makes meal prepping slightly more difficult, but at least you'll make sure everyone eats what they like.

When shopping for ingredients you also need to consider how many meals you are going to prepare. The more meals, the more it pays to buy in bulk.

You can do your shopping on a Friday afternoon on your way home from work, or anytime during the week or weekend if that suits your lifestyle. However, if you're not used to cooking large quantities of food, you may start by cooking for only two days ahead until you become better-organized.

THE ESSENTIAL TIPS FOR PREPARING MEALS

Meal prepping starts with meal planning and food shopping. The tricky part starts when you get home and have to organize all the ingredients, prepare them, cook them, and finally store them to be used at a later date. The very thought of having to spend several hours cooking for a week ahead may be enough to put people off the meal prepping idea. If you are new to this, the first thing you should do when you get home and unload all the food on your countertop is to have a cup of herbal tea (that surely will calm you down).

Change into more comfortable clothes, put on some nice music, and you're ready to start. Then, if you haven't done so already, clean out your fridge and throw out all the foods that are beyond the "use by" date. Clean the fridge if you need to.

Put the perishables and foods you will not be cooking that day in the fridge as soon as you get home, e.g. lettuce, fruits, etc. Besides, you should try to avoid as many distractions while you're cooking as that will only prolong the time you spend in the kitchen (e.g. don't read your emails or SMSs, don't even answer the phone, etc.).

Once you're ready, start cleaning, rinsing, chopping, grating, boiling, and sorting. When meal prepping becomes a routine, it won't take a lot of time.

There's something else to consider. Our thoughts affect our emotions and behavior and according to Ayurveda, it's particularly important not to be in a bad mood when cooking. To those who are not familiar with the philosophy of Ayurveda, this may come as a surprise, but most women will confirm that, if possible, you should refrain from cooking or baking if feeling resentful, angry, stressed, or exhausted. They may not have heard of Ayurveda but they know that emotions and thoughts DO affect the final result.

Why do I mention this? If you have to cook for a big family or family members with different diets and preferences and you are the only one who has to do the shopping, cooking, and cleaning afterward, you may often feel unappreciated. The trouble is that the resentment and bitterness which you are unaware of may find its way to your meals. I know that might sound cheeky but it is what it is. When feeling this way, either ask someone else to do the cooking or postpone the cooking for another day when your mind is not flooded with negative thoughts.

MEAL PREPPING WORKFLOW

Meal prepping starts with preparing ingredients for different meals. The more meals you plan to prepare, the better organized you need to be when it comes to shopping, cooking, and storing. What helps is preparing meals in a specific order.

A well-thought-through workflow can save you a lot of time. Choose which meals to cook first based on cook times. Before you start cooking, check if you have all the ingredients you had planned to use that day. You should have selected recipes beforehand, i.e. before you have done the shopping.

Once prepared, meals should be cooled and stored in the fridge, if you plan to use them in the next couple of days or the freezer if you plan on using them at a much later date.

TIPS FOR A WELL-ORGANIZED WORKFLOW:

- Slow Cooker first

Start with meals that require the longest cook time. Although food cooked in slow cookers takes a long time to cook, cooking this way saves you time because if your cooker has an automatic timer, all you have to do is set it to a certain time. Foods cooked "low and slow" also tend to retain more nutrients. However, cooking in a slow cooker may take as long as 8 hours, so if cooking in bulk, it's best to start with a meal that should be cooked this way. While it cooks, you have plenty of time to cook all the other meals you had planned for that day.

- Oven-cooked recipes next

An oven needs some time to reach the desired temperature and although meals cooked in the oven generally taste better than those cooked on the stovetop, they usually take longer to cook. This is why they should be done immediately after the slow cooker meals. Or, if you are not using a slow cooker, start by preparing the meal that needs to be cooked in the oven first.

- Stove Top recipes next

Once the slow-cooker and oven-cooked meals are underway, you can focus on meals cooked on the stovetop, which is where most of the meals are prepared. Meals that are only partly cooked and that will be cooked at a later date may take as little as 10 minutes of cook time. Others that need to be cooked thoroughly, will take an hour or so.

- No-Bake recipes next

Cold meals are usually done last and you can start with them only once other meals are cooking or have already been cooked and are cooling.

- Putting it all together

To make it easier to stick to the Dr. Sebi Alkaline Diet plan, start meal prepping so that you always have Dr. Sebi approved meals ready even if you don't feel like cooking or come home too late to start cooking from scratch. Besides, don't forget that Dr. Sebi's diet includes many herbs and herbal teas. When shopping for ingredients to use in your meals, make sure you don't run out of herbs and spices.

The meal prep basics revolve around preparing meals ahead of time and storing them in a way that will preserve their nutrients, flavor, and color. To achieve this, certain rules need to be followed.

CONTAINERS

Healthy food stored in the wrong way or wrong containers is a waste of time and money. As meal prepping is cooking for a few days or weeks, ahead, such meals are usually frozen or kept in the fridge. Either way, you need containers to keep the food in. Many different types of containers are available today and they come with different advantages, storage capacities, and prices. As proper storage can affect how a meal keeps and how it tastes, it's very important to choose containers that will help improve the taste rather than ruin it. But, before you go shopping for containers, make sure you know what you're going to use them for, e.g. for reheating, deep-freezing, pantry storage, etc.

11 COMMON TYPES OF CONTAINERS:

1. Grab-and-go containers
2. Glass containers
3. Stainless steel containers
4. BPA-free containers
5. Stackable containers
6. Leakproof containers
7. Dishwasher-safe/Oven-safe containers
8. Microwave-safe containers
9. Freezer-safe containers
10. Compartmentalized containers
11. Airtight containers

Another thing to consider when choosing containers is if you need reusable or single-use ones. Besides, containers are made from different materials which range from simple food plastic bags to sturdy ones made of plastic, silicone, or stainless steel. However, most containers are made of plastic and if you are environmentally conscious, you can get some eco-friendly ones made from stainless steel, glass, or bamboo. Personally, I like to go for over-safe glass containers. Although they are pricey, the value you get from the investment is worth every penny. Another thing to consider is the shape and size. If you plan to store a huge amount of food or if you have very little freezing space, stackable containers would probably be the best. Alternatively, get some simple plastic food bags.

BASIC FOOD STORAGE GUIDELINES

How tasty and healthy your frozen meals are will depend not only on the ingredients used and your cooking methods but also on the way they were stored. Proper storage helps your meals retain as much of their natural flavor and nutrients as possible. So, knowing how to prepare meals is only half the job. They also need to be stored, frozen, defrosted, and reheated correctly. How long foods can be kept in a fridge or a freezer before their nutrients are affected depends on the type of food, but also on how they were processed. However, even deep-frozen foods cannot stay frozen indefinitely.

ALKALINE VEGAN COLD FOOD STORAGE CHART

Produce	Optimal storage temp (F)	Optimal storage temp C	Storage Life
Apples	30-40	-1 -4	1-12 months
Avocado, ripe	38-45	+3 - +7	
Avocado, unripe	45-50	+7 - +10	
Burro bananas, green	62-70	17 – 21	
Burro bananas, ripe	56-60	13 – 16	
Basil	52-59	11 – 15	
Beans, dry	40-50		6 – 10 months
Beans, green	40-45		7 – 10 days
Blackberries	32-33	0 – 1	2-3 days
Blueberries	32-35	0 – 2	
Cantaloupe	36-38	2 – 3	
Cherries, sour	32	0	3 – 7 days
Cherries, sweet	32	0	2 – 3 weeks

Cucumber	50-55		10 - 14 days
Currants	31-32		1-4 weeks
Lettuce	32	0	2-3 weeks
Figs	32-35	0 – 2	
Herbs	32-35	0 – 2	
Kale	32		2 – 3 weeks
Limes	48-55	9 – 13	
Mango	50-55	10 – 13	
Mushrooms	32	0	3 – 4 days
Peaches	31-32		2 – 4 weeks
Pears	29-31		2 – 7 months
Plums	31-32		2 – 5 weeks
Prunes	31-32		2 – 5 weeks
Squash	41-50		1 – 2 weeks
Strawberries	32	0	3 – 7 days
Turnip greens	32		10 – 14 days
Watercress	32		2 – 3 weeks
Tomatillo	55-70		4 – 7 days

DETOX OR CLEANSING YOURSELF

WHAT IS A DETOX?

A Detox is a form of alternative medicine procedure that seeks to rid the body of toxins that have accumulated and that have unwanted effects on health. During detox cleanse, the body and most importantly, the digestive tract shuts down and this allows the body to focus more on healing because it's no longer using energy to aid and digestion. The amount of time that you cleanse helps a lot in the healing process, so the longer the fast, the better the results—but it is not the only factor for good results.

It's very important to cleanse at least once per year for 7 days if you are consuming an alkaline diet. However, if you are not eating an alkaline diet, you should cleanse at least every 2 to 3 months for at least 7 days.

TYPES OF DETOX

Detox can be done in several ways. The most common is through "fasting".

FASTING

There are several types of fasting you can choose to do and your choice will depend on several factors including the type of illness, your level of toxification, and your body tolerance level. Below are the types you can choose from ranging from liquid to solid fast.

- Water Fast
- Liquid Fast (Juice)
- Smoothie Fast
- Fruit fast
- Raw food fast (Veggies)

Dr. Sebi recommends fasting for at least 12 days on Spring water, sea moss, herbs, fruit, and alkaline juice. During the detox/Cleanse Stage, you can use the following to detox:

- Herbs
- Irish sea moss
- Spring water
- Alkaline fruit juices
- Alkaline Green juices
- Alkaline smoothies
- Tamarind

Note that all the above must be listed in the Dr. Sebi's food list. The body must be cleaned on an intra-cellular level through detox. This will ensure each cell is purified and free from mucus and toxins. Dr. Sebi recommends a total body cleanse to rid the body of disease—regardless of what type of disease, since he said only one disease exists. That means, to rid the body of disease, we must cleanse all organs of the body including the liver, kidney, colon, gall bladder, skin, and lymph glands.

HOW TO DO A NATURAL DETOX CLEANSE

There are several ways that you can detox, but the most commonly recognized way is through fasting. There are various types of fast which include:

- Water fast: In the water fast, you are expected to consume only spring water during a specified time of the detox/cleanse phase.
- Liquid fast: This is basically a fast on liquids except water. Liquids such as fruit juices, veggie juices and tamarind come in handy. To juice a fruit or vegetable, simply blend up a fruit or veggie and use a juicer to extract the juice.
- Fruit fast: This basically is a fast on fruits only.
- Raw Veggie fast: Fast on raw veggies which you'll have to consume raw.

WATER FAST

When performing the water type fast, you'll only drink spring water while taking your cleansing herbs and sea moss. Nothing else should be consumed for the duration of the fast. During the water fast, you should consume your cleansing herbs alongside and they can be taken either in tea or capsule form. Usually, it is recommended to do a detox fast for 7 to 14 days, so you can do a water fast for at least 7 days. However, note that how long you choose to do your water fast would depend a lot on your state of health, the level of toxicity in your body system and your tolerance level.

If you feel you are unable to do a water fast or maybe have any underlying health issues that may make water fast impossible or unsustainable, then you can instead choose a fruit fast or a raw veggie smoothie fast. The fruit or raw veggie fast can be taken either in juice, smoothie or whole form.

LIQUID FAST (JUICE)

Another fantastic way to fast is on liquids, also juices. Juices include all fruit and vegetable juices as well as tamarind juice. To juice a fruit or vegetable, simply blend up a fruit or veggie and use a juicer to extract the juice. Of course, while fasting on juices, you should also take your cleansing herbs alongside.

SMOOTHIE FAST

If you choose a smoothie fast, you should only drink smoothies prepared from fruits or vegetables. So, you can do either a fruit smoothie or a vegetable smoothie. Although it is recommended to fast for 7 to 14 days, you can actually fast longer on smoothies. This is especially if your body system is able to tolerate it. However, I recommend fasting for at least 14 days even though our healer Dr. Sebi himself fasted for 90 days on tamarind juice, spring water, and cleansing herbs.

FRUIT FAST

For fruit fast, it is expected that you consume only fruits. The fruits you consume can range from a variety of high-water content to soft massed fruits listed on the Dr. Sebi Nutritional guide. Again, how long you do this type of fast would depend on your tolerance levels.

HOW MUCH CLEANSING HERBS TO TAKE ON DETOX?

Just like every other alternative treatment, you should be mindful of the particular dosages to take when starting your detox. But one common problem with herbal remedies is the difficulty in determining the actual dosage to consume especially with raw herbs or roots. However, these have been made much easier with herbs that come in powder or granulated forms. With this, it's easier to make herbal teas with specific ratios.

However, for full form roots and herbs, I usually recommend researching the actual dosage amount to take. For pre-made herb packages, simply follow the manufacturer's dosage instructions. If they do not come with instructions, the general rule ratio to follow is 1 teaspoon part herb to 1 cup (8 ounces) of spring water. You can scale this ratio to make a larger volume so you can store it for use.

- For pre-purchase cleansing packages:
  Always follow the package recommended dosage or instructions on how you should prepare or take them. Most purchased packages come with instructions on how to take them.
- For Leafy purchased herbs:
  For leafy purchased herbs, research the particular dosage for the specific leafy herb you want to prepare.
- For bulk purchase herbs:
  If you have purchased herbs in bulk and you're making your own teas, find out what the proposed dosage is for each herb. As a general rule, you should prepare each herbal tea in a ratio of 1 teaspoon to 8 ounces of spring water.
- For capsules:
  For herbs that come in capsule form, you should follow the recommended dosages for each herbal capsule.

HOW TO PREPARE CLEANSING HERBS?

Preparing your cleansing herbs would depend a lot on the form you purchased them. Although, it's easier to prepare cleansing herbs that come in powder forms, as you can easily make herbal teas with them in the specified or recommended dosage. However, for other forms form herbs especially roots or leaves, it is better to use a ratio of 1 teaspoon to 1 cup (8 oz) of spring water for each herb.

However, for easier batch preparation and storage, I recommend preparing herbs in batches of mixtures. That would mean mixing them up according to function and benefit. Again, this will depend on what state of health and what minerals are most important for you. You can combine similar herbs with similar functions into a batch. Like our healer, Dr. Sebi would say, "If you want calcium, you know where to go to (sea moss), if you want Iron, you go to Burdock, and if you want a mix of both Iron and Fluorine, you go to Lily of the Valley."

In all, try not to mix more than 2 or 3 herbs together. Remember, these herbs are electric, and it's best to preserve their organic carbon, hydrogen and oxygen nature as much as we can. Again, if you mix more than that, you may not get their accurate concentrations per ml of water, so try to limit it to 3, possibly 2.

For a clearer understanding, you can use the following mix:

- o   Mix Colon and gallbladder cleansing herbs together
- o   Mix liver and kidney cleansing herbs
- o   Mix respiratory and mucus cleansing herbs
- o   Mix lymphatic and heavy-metal cleansing herbs.

Since these herbs perform a whole-body cleanse (not just colon) including the skin, eyes, colon, liver, lymphatic system, and gallbladder, you can decide to choose how to combine them. Also, note that when you make larger batches of these herbs for storage, try not to make batches that last more than 7 to 14 days

1.   For pre-purchase cleansing packages
   Please follow the recommended dosage or instructions that are provided for that cleansing package
2.   For fresh Green leafy herbs

a.   Place in spring water and boil on low heat for 5 to 7 min

b.   For dried leafy herbs, boil longer—10 to 15 min

3.   For Dried ground (or powder) herbs

For dried ground or powder leaves or roots, mix in recommended ratios for the herb. Powder herbs are the easiest to mix in dosage proportions so you can simply follow the package instructions

4.   For Chunks of Dried Root herbs

If you've purchased chunks of roots or stems, you can prepare them in the following way:

1.   Cut or break up chunks

2.   Place in spring water and boil for 15 minutes

3.   Let cool and serve

4.   Alternatively, prepare in larger batches and place in jars to store in the refrigerator.

5.   For bulk purchase herbs

If you have purchased herbs in bulk and you're making your own teas, find out what the recommended dosage is for each herb. As a general rule, you should prepare each herbal tea in a ratio of 1 teaspoon to 8 ounces of spring water.

6.   For capsules

I recommend that you do research and find out what the recommended dosage is for each herbal capsule

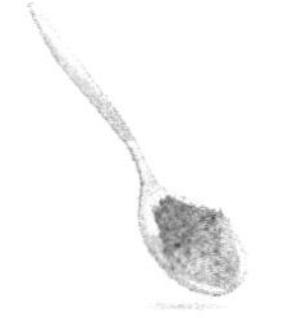

**1 teaspoon
Herb**

+

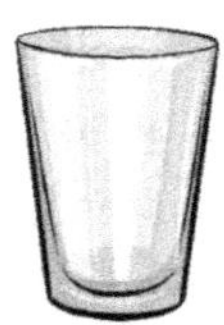

**1 Cup (8 oz)
Spring water**

HOW TO TAKE THE PREPARED CLEANSING HERBS

If you are on medication, I recommend that you take the herbs one hour before taking your meds this was actually recommended by Dr. Sebi. Your colon cleansing herbs should not be consumed for longer than 30 days because your body may become dependent on them and you want to start to reduce the dose during your last 3 to 5 days depending on how long you've been taking them.

ROUTINE

- Twice a day—morning and night
- Daily Consistency—Try to stay consistent both in terms of timing and duration. That is, try not to skew the duration. Make it consistent and take the cleansing herb throughout the duration of the cleanse. For example, for a 14-day cleanse, the cleansing herbs can be taken twice daily, and you should take them around the same time you do take them on both mornings and evenings.

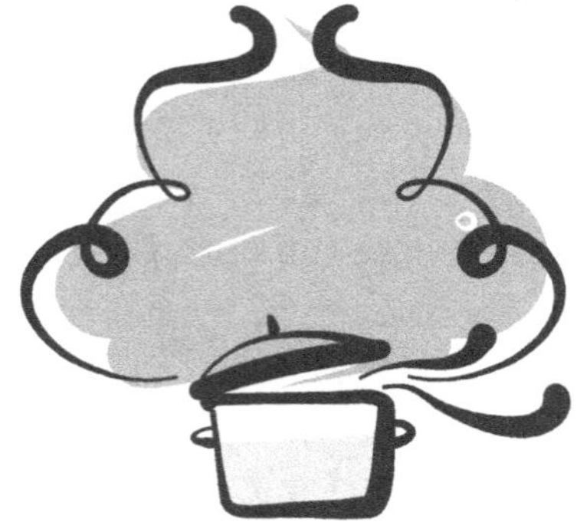

THE BREAKFASTS

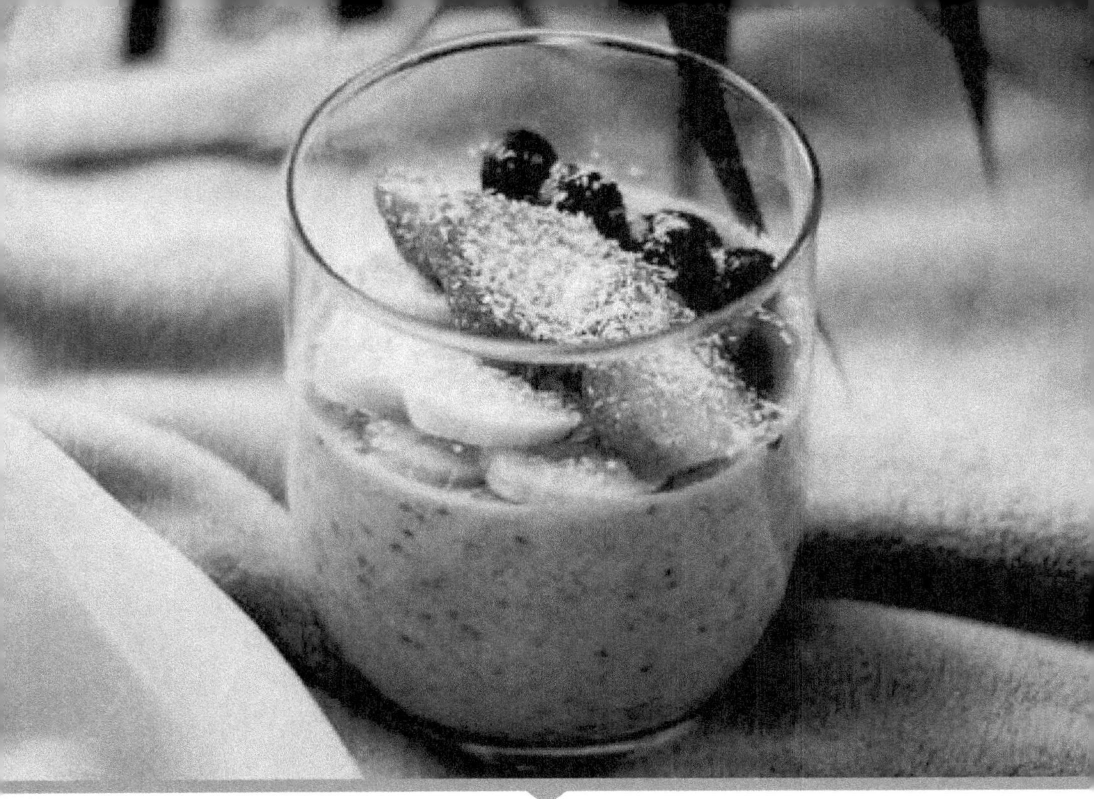

1. STRAWBERRY AND CHIA SEED OVERNIGHT OATS PARFAIT

Preparation Time: 10 Minutes

Cooking Time: 0 Minutes

Servings: 1 or 2

INGREDIENTS:

For the Strawberry Mixture

- 1 cup diced strawberries
- 1 teaspoon chia seeds
- 1 to 2 teaspoons brown rice syrup

For the Oat Mixture

> 1 cup quick rolled oats
> 1 cup coconut milk (boxed)
> 1 tablespoon brown rice syrup
> ⅛ tablespoon vanilla bean powder

DIRECTIONS:

To Prepare the Strawberry Mixture

1. In a small bowl, stir together the strawberries, chia seeds, and brown rice syrup until well combined.

To Prepare the Oat Mixture

2. In a small bowl, stir together the oats, coconut milk, brown rice syrup, and vanilla bean powder until well combined.
3. Place half the oat mixture in the bottom of 1 large glass mason jar or 2 small jars, and layer half of the strawberry mixture over the oat mixture. Repeat with the remaining oat and strawberry mixtures.
4. Cover the mason jar(s), and refrigerate overnight.
5. Uncover and enjoy.

NUTRITION:

Calories: 238
Total Fat: 21g
Total Carbohydrates: 15g
Fiber: 6g
Sugar: 6g
Protein: 2g

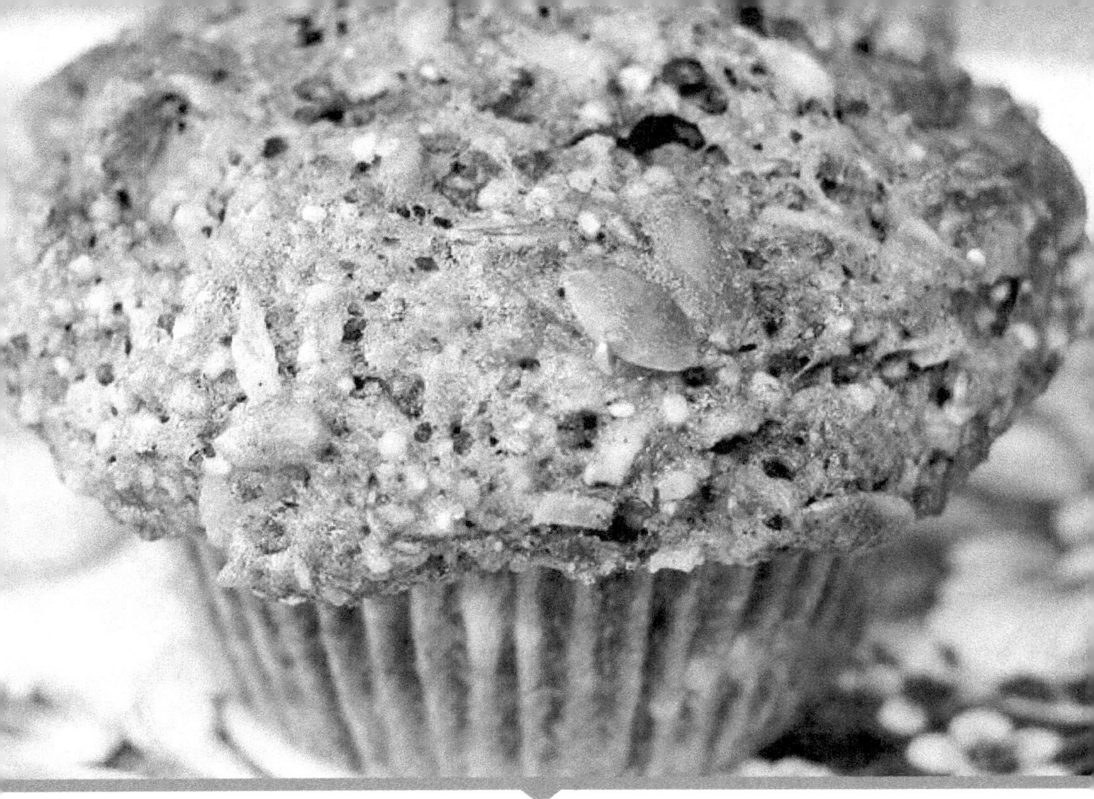

2.   CARROT AND HEMP SEED MUFFINS

Preparation Time: 5 Minutes

Cooking Time: 25 Minutes

Servings: 12

INGREDIENTS:

- 3 tablespoons water
- 1 tablespoon ground flaxseed
- 2 cups oat flour
- 1 cup almond milk (boxed)
- ½ cup unrefined whole cane sugar, such as Sucanat
- 1 carrot, shredded
- 6 tablespoons cashew butter
- 2 tablespoons hemp seeds

- ➢ 1 tablespoon chopped lacinato kale
- ➢ 1 tablespoon baking powder
- ➢ ⅛ teaspoon vanilla bean powder
- ➢ Pinch sea salt

DIRECTIONS:

1. Preheat the oven to 350°F.
2. To prepare a flax egg, in a small bowl, whisk together the water and flaxseed.
3. Transfer the flax egg to a medium bowl, and add the oat flour, almond milk, sugar, carrot, cashew butter, hemp seeds, kale, baking powder, vanilla bean powder, and salt, stirring until well combined.
4. Divide the mixture evenly among 12 muffin cups, bake for 20 to 25 minutes, and enjoy right away.

NUTRITION:

Calories: 330
Total Fat: 10g
Total Carbohydrates: 49g
Fiber: 20g
Sugar: 8g
Protein: 17g

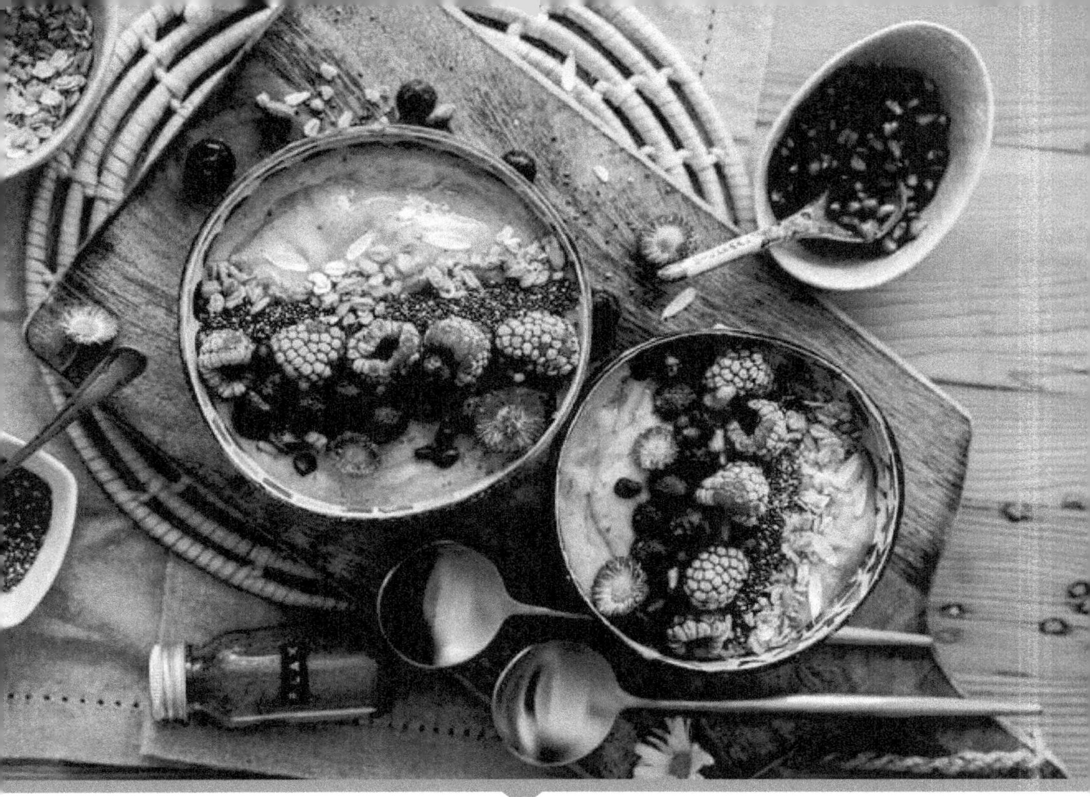

3.   RASPBERRY-AVOCADO SMOOTHIE BOWL

Preparation Time: 5 Minutes

Cooking Time: 0 Minutes

Servings: 2

INGREDIENTS:

- 1½ cups coconut milk (boxed)
- 1 cup raspberries, plus more (optional) for topping
- 1 avocado, roughly chopped
- 3 tablespoons unrefined whole cane sugar, such as Sucanat, divided
- 1 teaspoon chia seeds
- 1 teaspoon unsweetened shredded coconut
- Mixed berries, for topping (optional)

▍ DIRECTIONS:

1. In a blender, blend to combine the coconut milk, raspberries, avocado, and 2 tablespoons of sugar until smooth and creamy.
2. Pour the mixture into 2 serving bowls, sprinkle the extra raspberries (if using), the remaining 1 tablespoon of the sugar, and the chia seeds, shredded coconut, and mixed berries (if using) over the top, and enjoy.

▍ NUTRITION:

Calories: 295
Total Fat: 19g
Total Carbohydrates: 24g
Fiber: 11g
Sugar: 3g
Protein: 7g

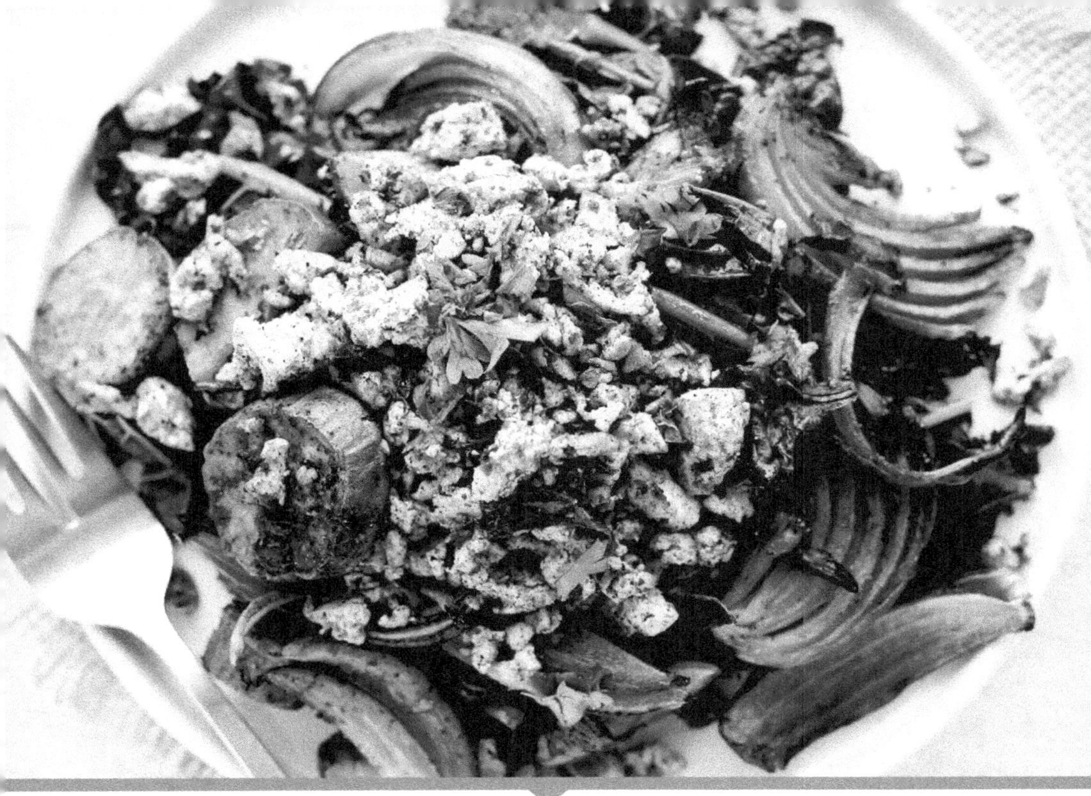

4. SWEET POTATO AND KALE BREAKFAST HASH

Preparation Time: 10 Minutes

Cooking Time: 15 Minutes

Servings: 1 or 2

❚ INGREDIENTS:

- ➤ 1 teaspoon avocado oil
- ➤ 2 cups peeled and cubed sweet potatoes
- ➤ ½ cup chopped kale
- ➤ ½ cup diced onion
- ➤ ½ teaspoon sea salt
- ➤ ½ teaspoon freshly ground black pepper

> ½ avocado, cubed (optional)
> 1 to 2 teaspoons sesame seeds or hemp seeds (optional)

DIRECTIONS:

1. In a large skillet over medium heat, heat the avocado oil. Add the sweet potatoes, kale, onion, salt, and pepper, and sauté for 10 to 15 minutes, or until the sweet potatoes are soft. Remove from the heat.
2. Gently stir in the avocado and sesame seeds (if using), transfer to 1 large or 2 small plates, and enjoy.

NUTRITION:

Calories: 230
Total Fat: 1g
Total Carbohydrates: 53g
Fiber: 10g
Sugar: 9g
Protein: 6g

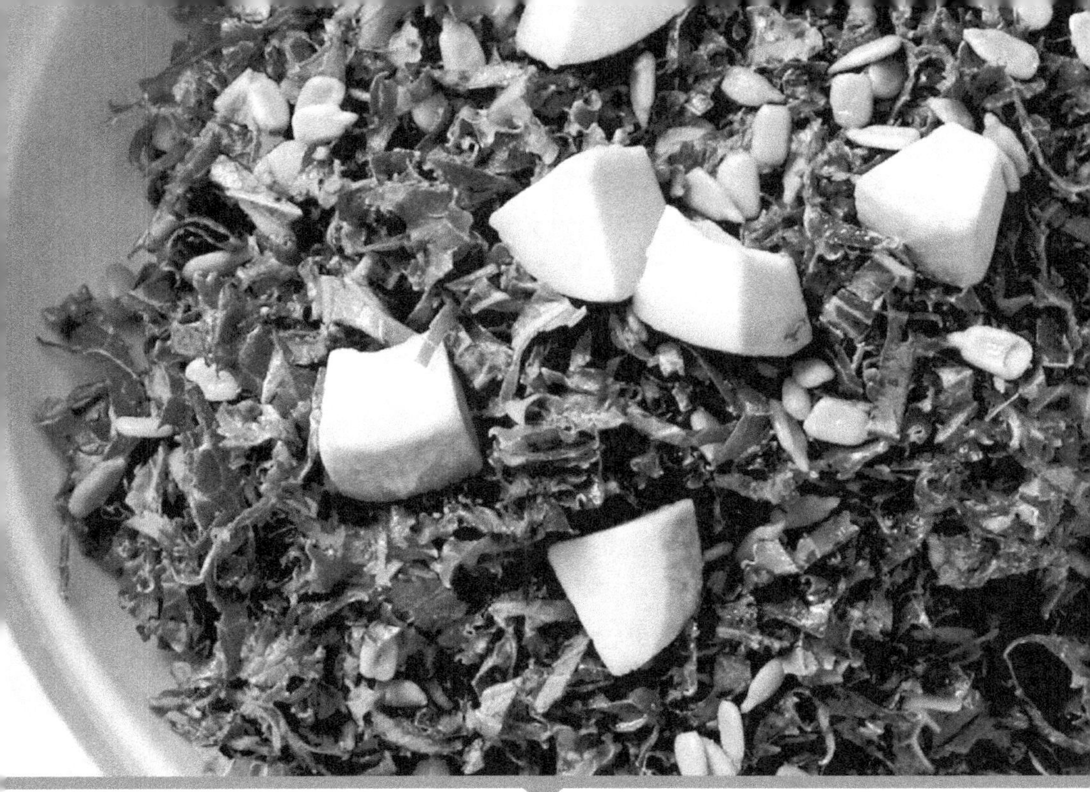

5. AVOCADOS WITH KALE AND ALMOND STUFFING

Preparation Time: 5 Minutes

Cooking Time: 0 Minutes

Servings: 1 or 2

INGREDIENTS:

- ½ cup almonds
- ½ cup chopped Lacinato kale
- 1 garlic clove
- ½ jalapeño
- 2 tablespoons nutritional yeast
- 1 tablespoon avocado oil

- ➤ 1 tablespoon apple cider vinegar
- ➤ 1 tablespoon freshly squeezed lemon juice
- ➤ ¼ teaspoon sea salt
- ➤ 1 avocado, halved and pitted

DIRECTIONS:

1. In a food processor, pulse the almonds, kale, garlic, jalapeño, nutritional yeast, avocado oil, apple cider vinegar, lemon juice, and sea salt until everything is well combined, the almonds are in small pieces, and it has a chunky texture, taking care not to overprocess.
2. Add half of the stuffing mixture to the center of each avocado half, and enjoy.

NUTRITION:

Calories: 295
Total Fat: 19g
Total Carbohydrates: 24g
Fiber: 11g
Sugar: 3g
Protein: 7g

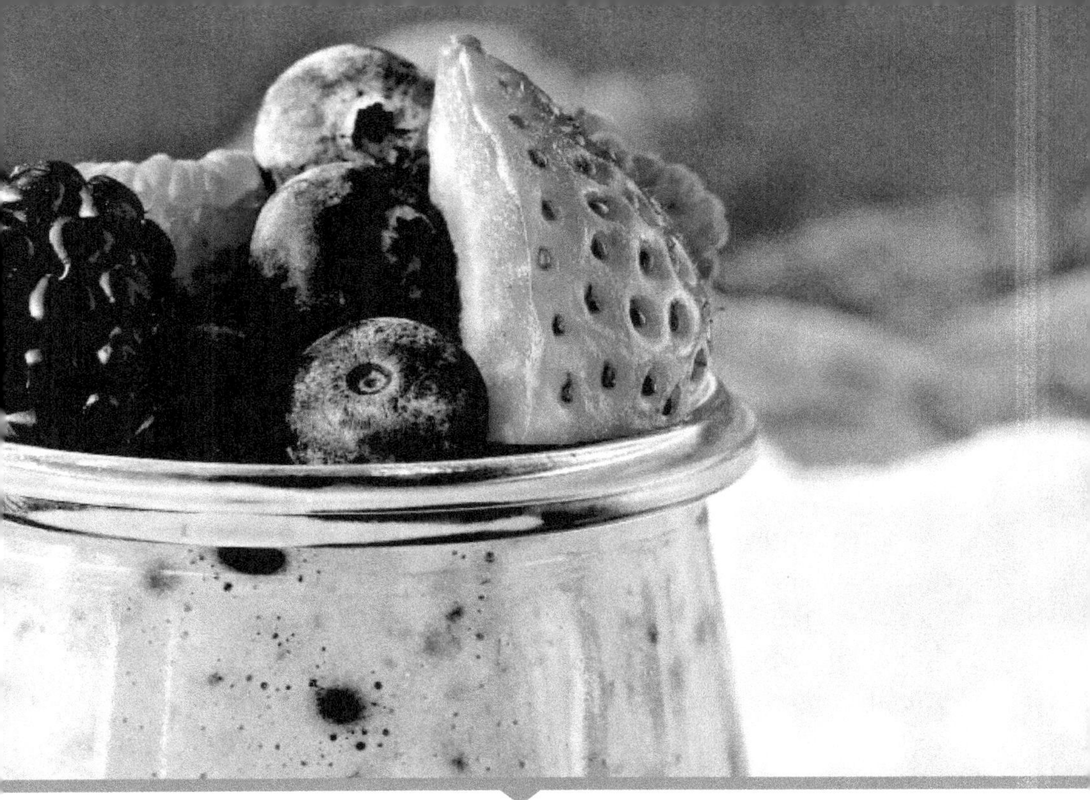

6. MIXED BERRY-CHIA SEED PUDDING

Preparation Time: 5 Minutes

Cooking Time: 0 Minutes

Servings: 1

INGREDIENTS:

- 1 cup coconut milk (boxed)
- ½ cup mixed berries (raspberries, blackberries, blueberries), plus more (optional) for topping
- 2 tablespoons chia seeds
- 1 to 2 tablespoons unrefined whole cane sugar, such as Sucanat

DIRECTIONS:

1. In a mason jar, combine the coconut milk, berries, chia seeds, and sugar, adjusting the sugar to your preference.
2. Seal the jar tightly, and shake vigorously until well mixed.
3. Refrigerate for about 1 hour, or until the pudding thickens to your preference.
4. Stir, top with the extra mixed berries (if using), and enjoy.

NUTRITION:

Calories: 345
Total Fat: 18g
Total Carbohydrates: 53g
Fiber: 26g
Sugar: 20g
Protein: 11g

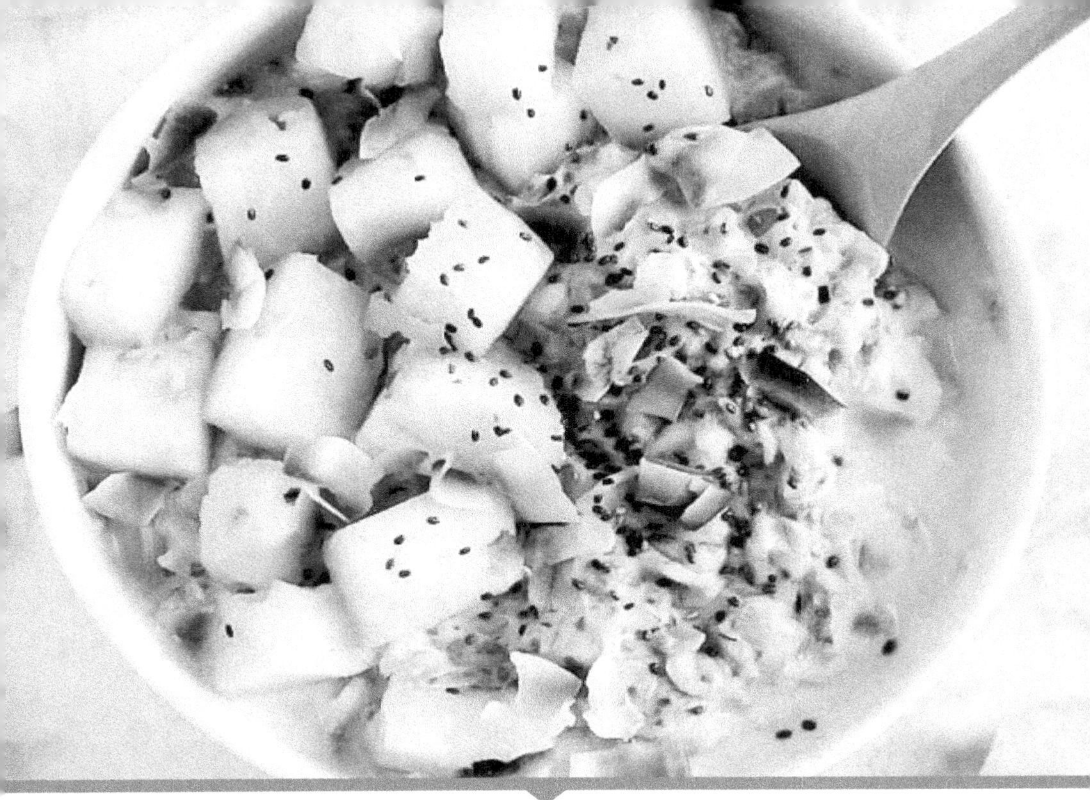

7. PINEAPPLE AND COCONUT OATMEAL BOWL

Preparation Time: 5 Minutes

Cooking Time: 5 Minutes

Servings: 2

INGREDIENTS:

For the oatmeal

- 1 cup quick rolled oats
- 1 (13.5-ounce) can full-fat coconut milk
- 2 tablespoons unrefined whole cane sugar, such as Sucanat

For assembling

- ½ cup cubed pineapple
- ¼ cup unsweetened coconut flakes
- 1 tablespoon chia seeds
- 1 tablespoon pumpkin seeds, chopped

DIRECTIONS:

To make the oatmeal

1. In a small saucepan over medium-low heat, cook the oats, coconut milk, and sugar for 3 to 5 minutes, or until the oats are soft; adjust the sugar to your preference.

To assemble

2. Transfer the oatmeal to 2 serving bowls, top with the cubed pineapple, coconut flakes, and chia and pumpkin seeds, and serve.

NUTRITION:

Calories: 370
Total Fat: 20g
Total Carbohydrates: 23g
Fiber: 10g
Sugar: 17g
Protein: 4g

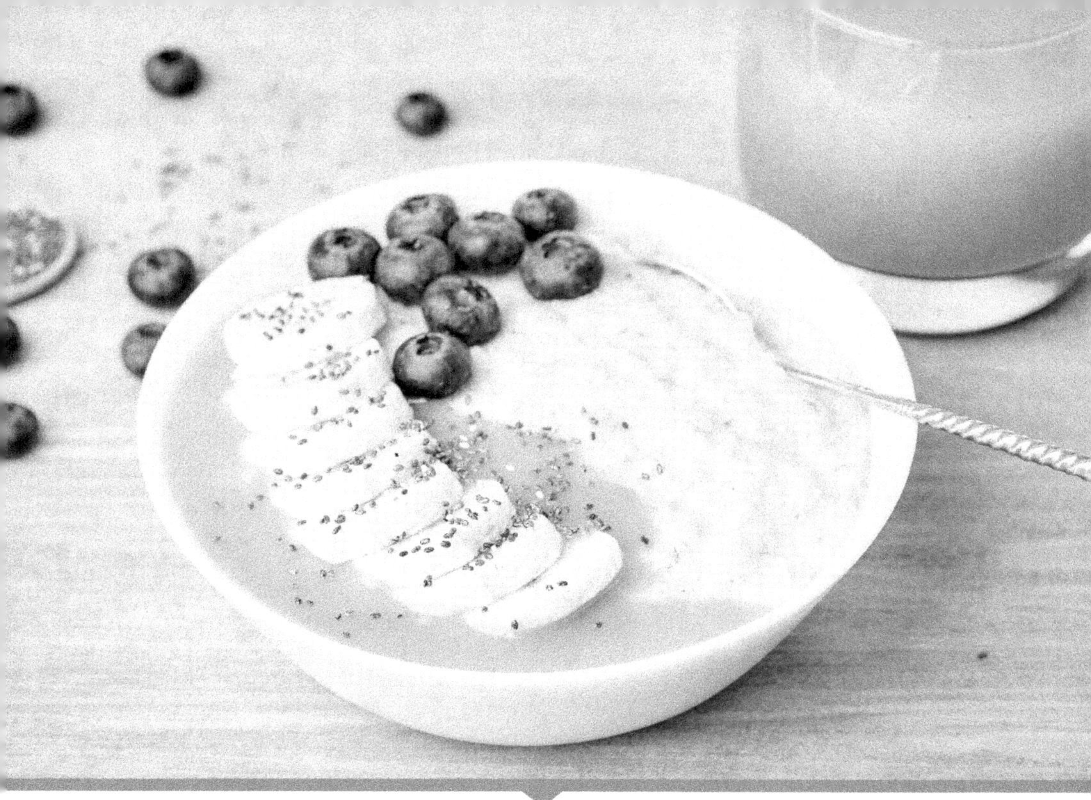

8. OATMEAL PORRIDGE WITH MANGO-CHIA FRUIT JAM

Preparation Time: 5 Minutes

Cooking Time: 5 Minutes

Servings: 2

INGREDIENTS:

- 1 (14-ounce) can full-fat coconut milk
- 1 cup quick rolled oats
- 2 tablespoons unrefined whole cane sugar, such as Sucanat
- 1 to 2 tablespoons mango Chia Seed Fruit Jam

▌ DIRECTIONS:

1. In a small saucepan over medium-low heat, cook the coconut milk, oats, and sugar, stirring occasionally, for 3 to 5 minutes, or until the oats are soft.
2. Transfer the oatmeal to 2 serving bowls, top with the mango Chia Seed Fruit Jam, and serve.

▌ NUTRITION:

Calories 265
Total Fat 18g
Total Carbohydrates 22g
Fiber 5g
Sugar 3g
Protein 5g

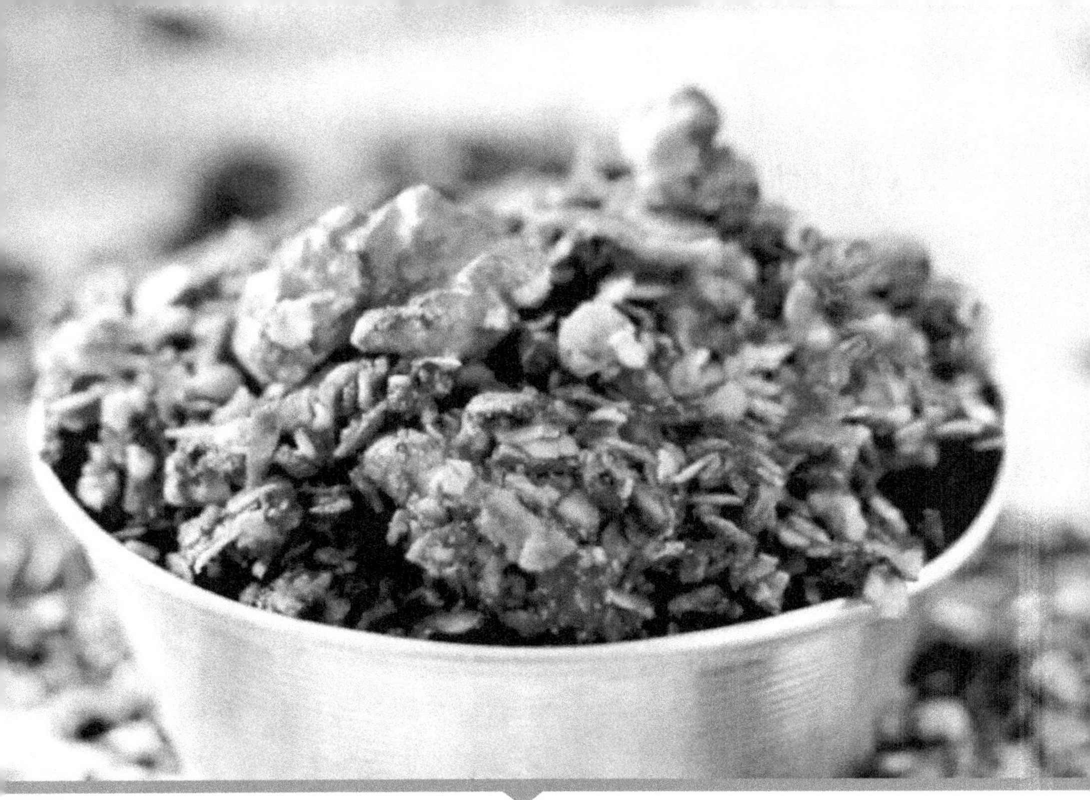

9. VANILLA BEAN AND CINNAMON GRANOLA

Preparation Time: 5 Minutes

Cooking Time: 30 Minutes

Servings: 3

INGREDIENTS:

- 3 cups quick rolled oats
- ½ cup brown rice syrup
- 6 tablespoons coconut oil
- ¼ cup unrefined whole cane sugar, such as Sucanat
- 2 teaspoons vanilla bean powder
- 2 teaspoons ground cinnamon
- ¼ teaspoon sea salt

DIRECTIONS:

1. Preheat the oven to 250° F. Line a baking pan with parchment paper.
2. In a large bowl, use your hands to mix together the oats, brown rice syrup, coconut oil, sugar, vanilla bean powder, cinnamon, and salt until well combined.
3. Squeeze the mixture together into a ball, and transfer to the prepared baking pan.
4. Press the mixture evenly on the baking pan, taking care not to break it up into small pieces. This will allow it to bake in large cluster pieces that you can break apart after baking, if you prefer.
5. Bake for about 30 minutes, or until crispy, taking care not to overbake.
6. Cool completely before serving. The granola will harden and get even crispier as it cools. Store in an airtight container.

NUTRITION:

Calories: 310
Total Fat: 30g
Total Carbohydrates: 12g
Fiber: 5g
Sugar: 3g
Protein: 6g

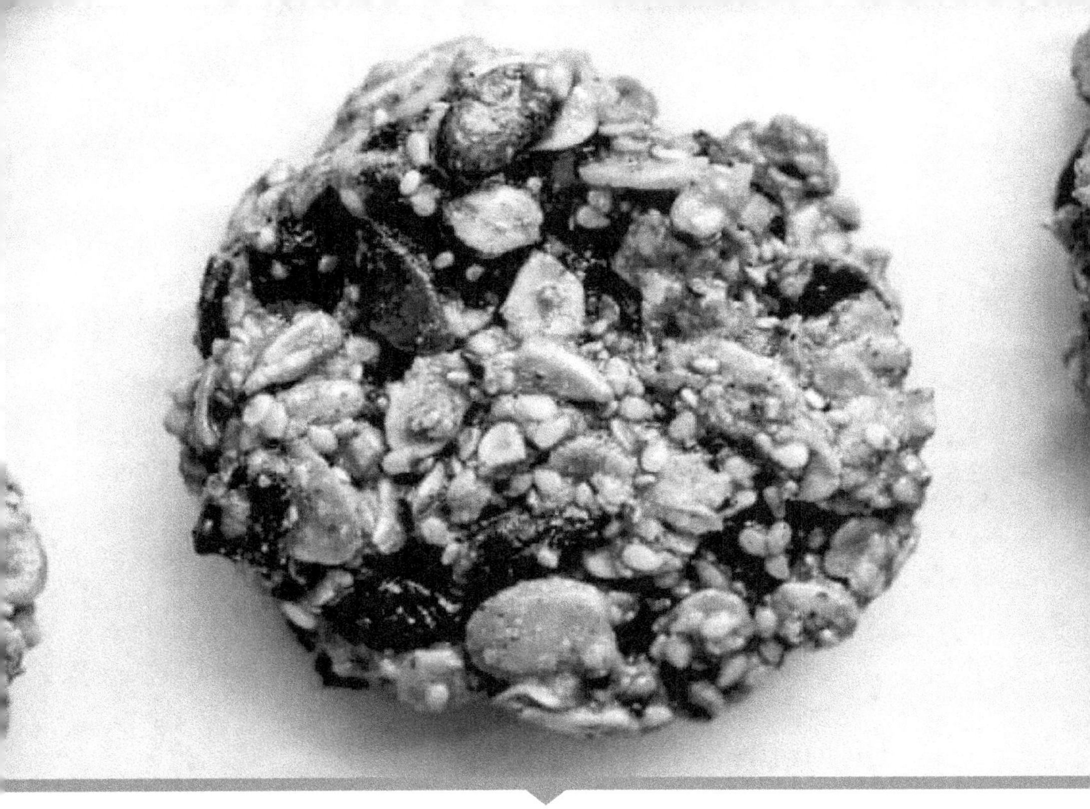

10. SESAME AND HEMP SEED BREAKFAST COOKIES

Preparation Time: 10 Minutes

Cooking Time: 0 Minutes

Servings: 15

INGREDIENTS:

- ⅔ cup cashew butter
- ½ cup quick rolled oats
- ¼ cup hemp seeds
- ¼ cup sesame seeds
- 3 tablespoons brown rice syrup
- 3 tablespoons coconut oil, melted

> ➢ 1 teaspoon vanilla bean powder
> ➢ 1 teaspoon ground cinnamon

DIRECTIONS:

1. Line a baking sheet with parchment paper.
2. In a medium bowl, stir together the cashew butter, oats, hemp seeds, sesame seeds, brown rice syrup, coconut oil, vanilla bean powder, and cinnamon until well combined.
3. Refrigerate the bowl for 5 to 10 minutes to allow the mixture to firm up.
4. Scoop a tablespoonful of dough at a time and flatten it into a disk with your hands. Smooth the outer edges with your fingertips, and place them on the prepared baking sheet. Repeat with the remaining dough.
5. Refrigerate the cookies for about 20 minutes, or until they firm up, and serve. Store leftovers in an airtight container in the refrigerator; they will soften and lose their shape at room temperature.

NUTRITION:

Calories: 800
Total Fat: 75g
Total Carbohydrates: 35g
Fiber: 28g
Sugar: 4g
Protein: 27g

11. FRESH FRUIT WITH VANILLA-CASHEW CREAM

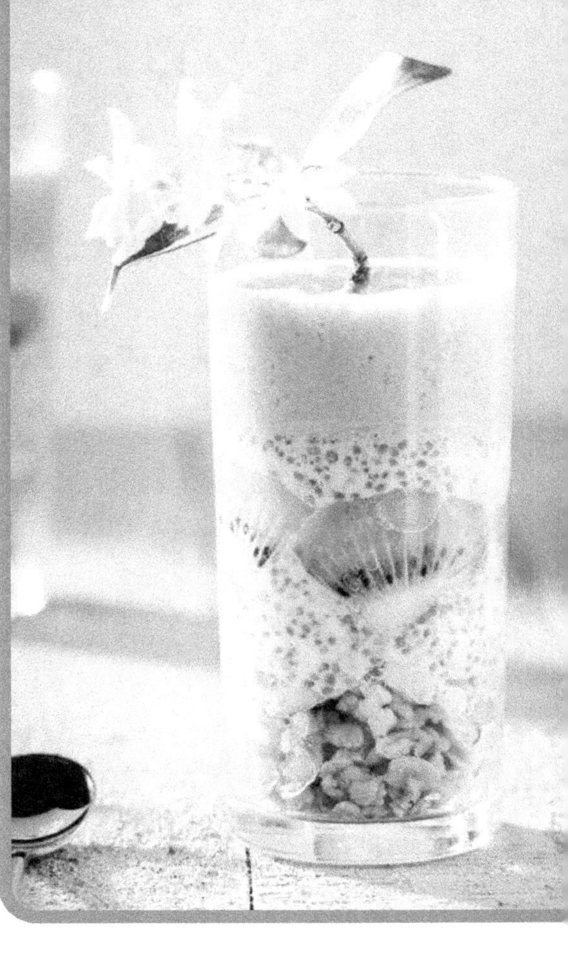

Preparation Time: 25 Minutes

Cooking Time: 0 Minutes

Servings: 4

INGREDIENTS:

- Room-temperature water, for soaking
- 1 cup raw cashews
- 1 (13.5-ounce) can coconut milk
- 2 tablespoons brown rice syrup
- 2 tablespoons unrefined whole cane sugar, such as Sucanat
- 2 teaspoons vanilla bean powder
- 1 teaspoon freshly squeezed lemon juice
- ¼ teaspoon ground cinnamon
- ¼ teaspoon sea salt
- 4 cups alkaline fruit, such as raspberries, blackberries, blueberries, strawberries, mango, pineapple, or cantaloupe

DIRECTIONS:

1. In a medium bowl with enough room-temperature water to cover them, soak the cashews for 15 to 20 minutes.
2. Drain and rinse the cashews.
3. In a high-speed blender, blend to combine the soaked cashews, coconut milk, brown rice syrup, sugar, vanilla bean powder, lemon juice, cinnamon, and salt until creamy and smooth. Add more sugar, if you like.
4. Add 1 cup of fruit to each of 4 serving bowls, drizzle each bowl of fruit with ½ cup of cream, and serve.

NUTRITION:

Calories: 160
Total Fat: 4g
Total Carbohydrates: 32g
Fiber: 4g
Sugar: 18g
Protein: 2g

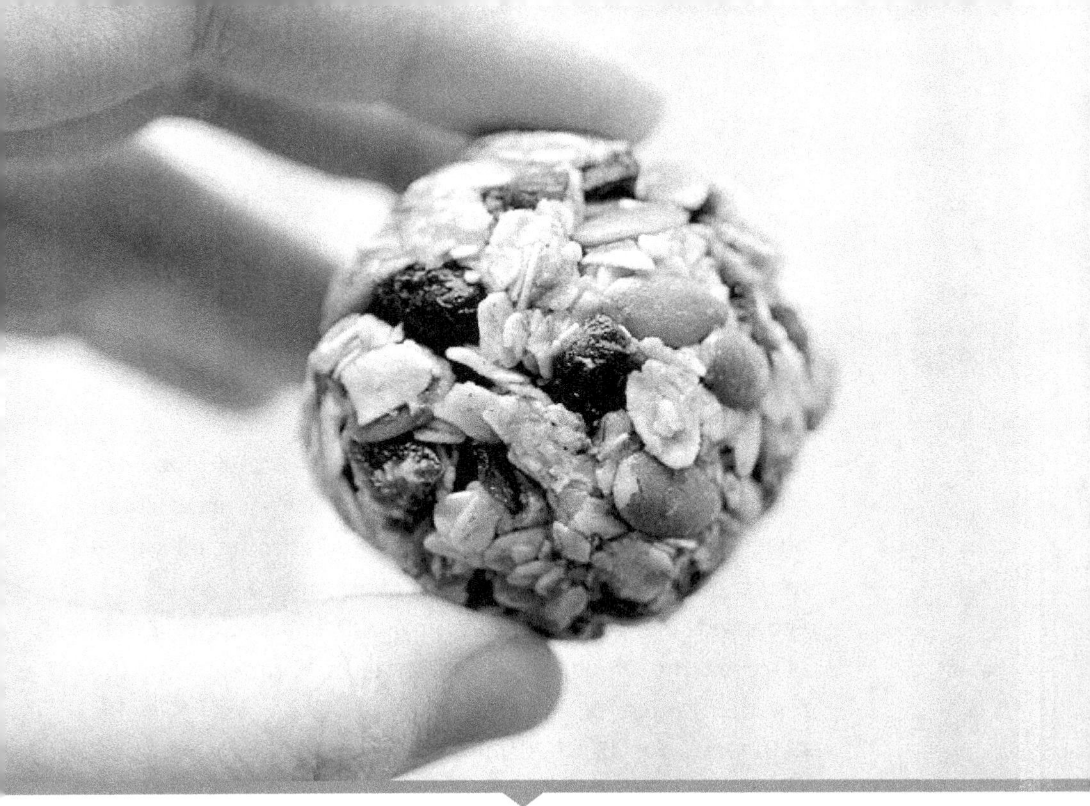

12. PUMPKIN SEED-PROTEIN BREAKFAST BALLS

Preparation Time: 5 Minutes

Cooking Time: 0 Minutes

Servings: 20

INGREDIENTS:

- 1½ cups quick rolled oats
- 3 tablespoons 100% organic pumpkin seed protein powder
- ½ cup almond butter
- ½ cup raw pumpkin seeds
- 3 tablespoons brown rice syrup
- 1 tablespoon coconut oil

- ➢ 1 teaspoon ground cinnamon
- ➢ 1 teaspoon vanilla bean powder
- ➢ 2 to 4 tablespoons coconut milk

▌DIRECTIONS:

1. Line a baking sheet with parchment paper.
2. In a food processor, process the oats, protein powder, almond butter, pumpkin seeds, brown rice syrup, coconut oil, cinnamon, vanilla bean powder, and coconut milk until well combined, taking care to not overprocess.
3. Scoop a tablespoonful into your hands and roll into a ball. Place on the prepared baking sheet, and repeat with the remaining mixture.
4. Refrigerate for 15 to 20 minutes, or until firm, and serve. Store in the refrigerator; the balls will get soft and lose their shape at room temperature.

▌NUTRITION:

Calories: 430
Total Fat: 3g
Total Carbohydrates: 71g
Fiber: 19g
Sugar: 8g
Protein: 22g

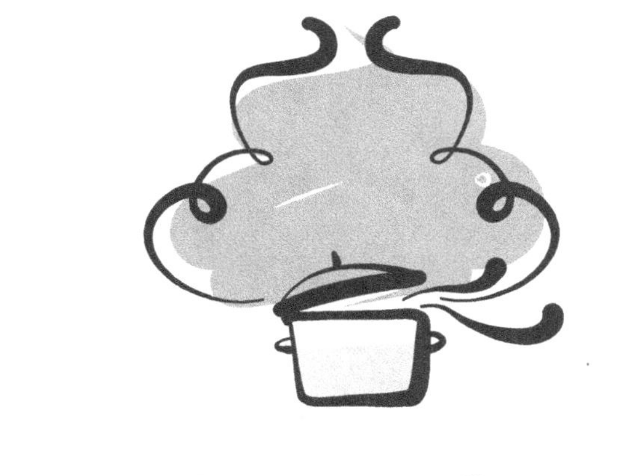

FIRST DISHES

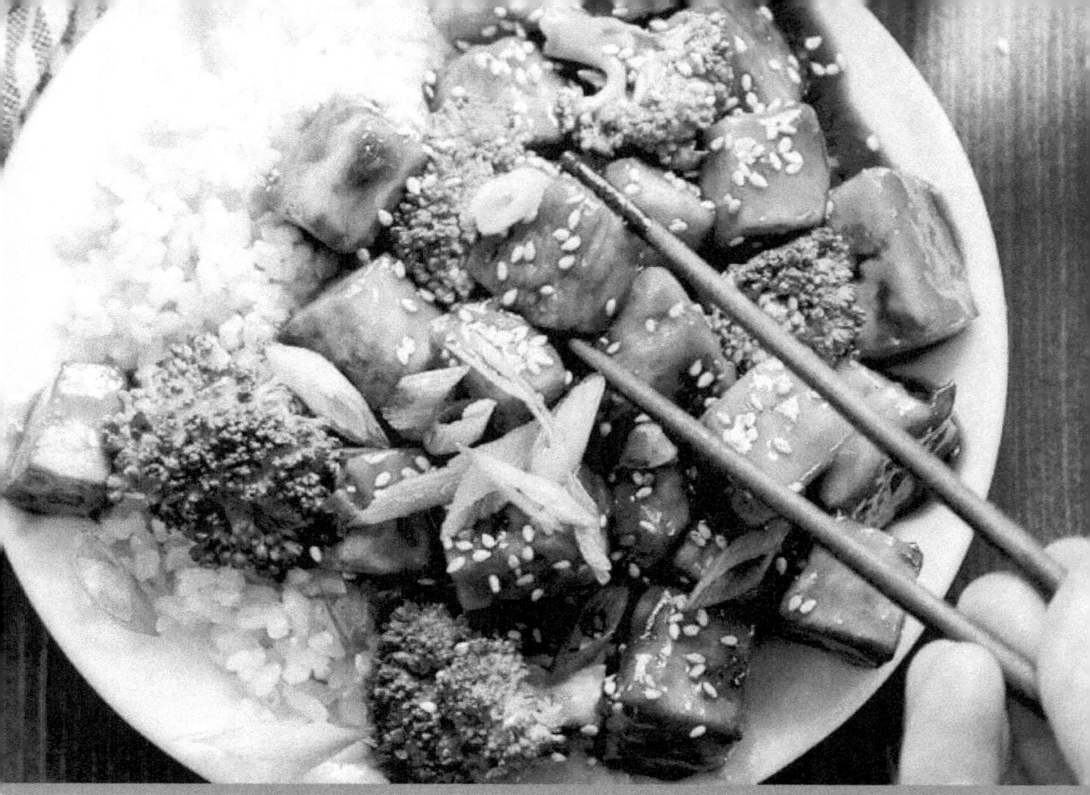

1.   TERIYAKI TOFU STIR-FRY

Preparation Time: 10 Minutes

Cooking Time: 20 Minutes

Servings: 4

INGREDIENTS:

For the Tofu:

- 2 tablespoons chopped green onions
- 2 cups asparagus
- 14 ounces (397 grams) tofu, firm, pressed
- 2 teaspoons red chili sauce
- 1 tablespoon soy sauce
- 3 teaspoons olive oil

For the Sauce:

- 2 tablespoons minced garlic
- 1 ½ tablespoons rice vinegar
- ½ tablespoon grated ginger
- 2 teaspoons corn starch
- ¼ cup (59 grams) coconut sugar
- 3 tablespoons soy sauce
- 1 tablespoon sesame oil
- ½ cup (118 ml) water

For Serving:

- 4 cups (946 grams) quinoa, cooked

DIRECTIONS:

1. Prepare the tofu: pat dry tofu and cut into ½-inch cubes.
2. Take a medium skillet pan, place it over medium-high heat, add 1 teaspoon oil and when hot, add tofu in a single layer, then cook for 3 to 4 minutes until golden brown.
3. Transfer tofu pieces to a large bowl, add 1 teaspoon oil in the pan and repeat with the remaining tofu cubes.
4. Meanwhile, prepare the sauce: take a small bowl, add all of the sauce ingredients in it and whisk until combined, then set aside until required.
5. When all the tofu gets cooked, drizzle them with sauces and toss until coated, set aside until required.
6. Wipe clean the skillet pan, return it over medium-high heat, add remaining oil and when hot, add asparagus and green onions, then cook for 3 minutes until tender-crisp.
7. Return tofu pieces into the pan, drizzle with prepared sauce, switch heat to medium level, toss until the ingredients are

well mixed, and cook for 3 to 5 minutes until the sauce starts to thicken.

8. When done, taste to adjust the seasoning of the sauce and then remove the pan from heat.

9. Distribute cooked quinoa among plates, top with tofu and vegetables, and then serve.

NUTRITION:

Cal: 11 g
Fat: 1 g
Saturated Fat: 58 g
Carbs: 8 g
Fiber: 19 g
Protein: 12 g

2. RED LENTIL AND QUINOA FRITTERS

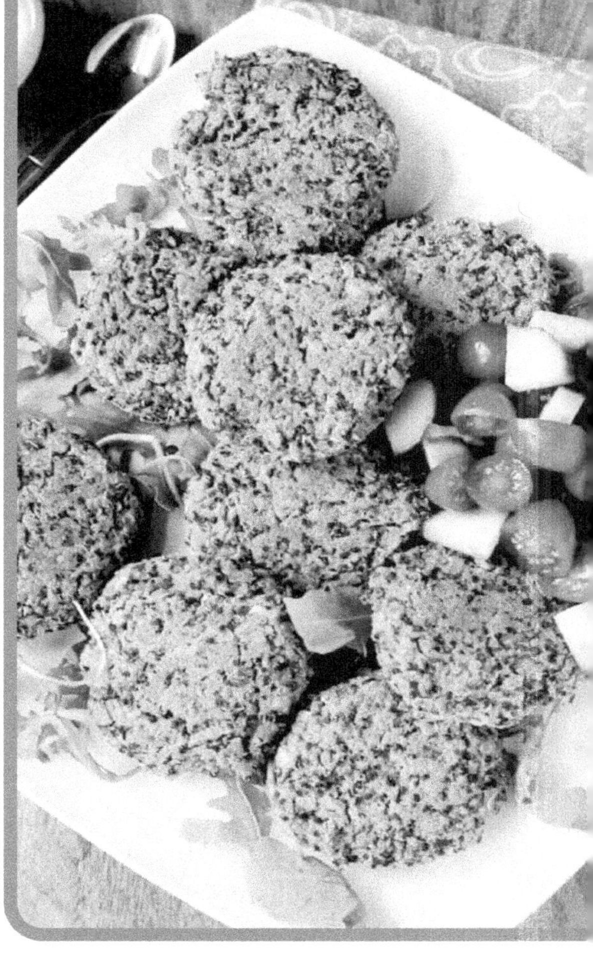

Preparation Time: 20 Minutes

Cooking Time: 25 Minutes

Servings: 10

INGREDIENTS:

For the Fritters:

- ¼ cup (59 grams) chickpea flour
- 1 ½ cups (354 grams) quinoa
- ¼ cup (59 grams) cornmeal
- ½ cup (118 grams) red lentils
- 2 teaspoons ground turmeric
- 1/8 teaspoon black bell pepper
- ½ teaspoon salt
- ¼ cup (59 grams) chopped parsley
- 1 teaspoon cumin
- ¼ teaspoon ground cinnamon
- ½ of a lemon, juiced
- 1 tablespoon Dijon mustard
- ¼ cup (59 grams) tahini
- 4 cups (946 ml) vegetable broth

For the Sauce:

- ➢ 1 teaspoon minced garlic
- ➢ ¼ teaspoon salt
- ➢ 1 tablespoon chopped dill
- ➢ 3 tablespoons tahini
- ➢ 1 lemon, juiced
- ➢ 1 cup coconut yogurt, unsweetened

DIRECTIONS:

1. Switch on the oven and set it to 400°F, and let it preheat.
2. Take a medium pot, place it over medium-high heat, add lentils and quinoa, pour in vegetable broth, and bring it to a boil.
3. Switch heat to medium-low level and simmer the grains for 15 minutes until cooked, covering the pot.
4. When done, let grains cool for 10 minutes, fluff them with a fork, and transfer them into a large bowl.
5. Add remaining ingredients for the fritters in it and stir well until incorporated.
6. Shape the mixture into ten patties, arrange them on a baking sheet lined with aluminum foil and bake until golden brown and thoroughly cooked, turning halfway.
7. Meanwhile, prepare the yogurt sauce: take a medium bowl, place all the ingredients for it inside and whisk until combined.
8. Serve fritters with yogurt sauce.

NUTRITION:

Cal: 173 g

Fat; 4 g

Saturated Fat: 1 g

Carbs: 27 g

Fiber: 2 g

Protein: 7 g

Sugar: 3 g

3. GREEN PEA FRITTERS

Preparation Time: 10 Minutes

Cooking Time: 25 Minutes

Servings: 4

INGREDIENTS:

For the Fritters:

- 1 ½ cups (140 grams) chickpea flour
- 2 cups (250 grams) frozen peas
- 1 large white onion, peeled, diced
- 1 tablespoon minced garlic
- 1/8 teaspoon salt
- 1 teaspoon baking soda
- 2 tablespoons mixed dried Italian herbs
- 1 tablespoon olive oil
- Water as needed

For the Yoghurt Sauce:

- ½ teaspoon dried rosemary
- ½ teaspoon dried parsley
- ½ teaspoon dried mint
- 1 lemon, juiced
- 1 cup of soy yogurt

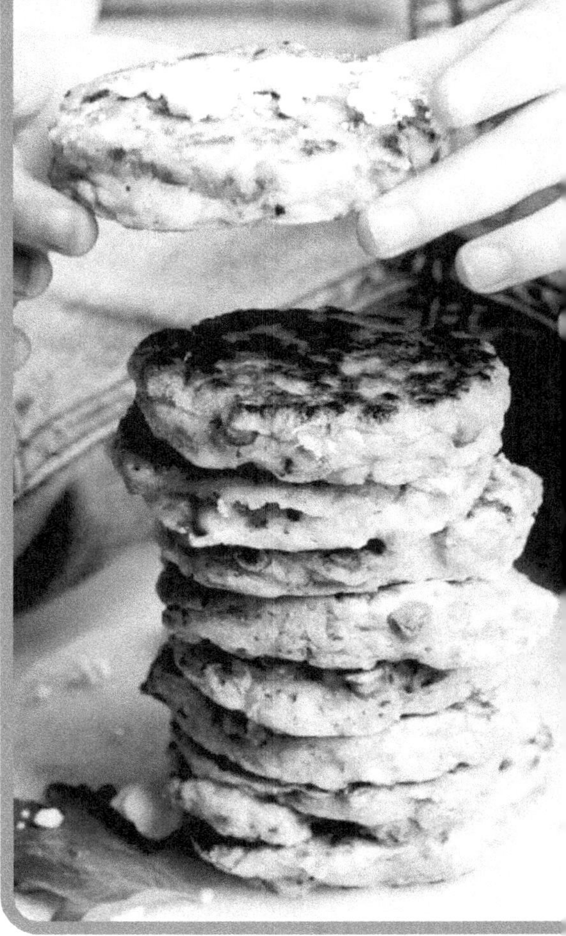

DIRECTIONS:

1. Preheat the oven for 350°F
2. Take a medium saucepan, place it over medium heat, add peas, cover them with water, bring it to a boil until tender, and when done, drain the peas and set aside until required.
3. Take a frying pan, place it over medium heat, add oil, and when hot, add onion and garlic; cook until softened.
4. Transfer onion-garlic mixture to a food processor, add peas and pulse for 1 minute until the thick paste comes together.
5. Tip the mixture in a bowl, add salt, baking soda, Italian herbs, and chickpea flour, stir until incorporated, and shape it into ten patties.
6. Brush the patties with oil, arrange them onto a baking sheet and bake for 15 to 18 minutes until golden brown and thoroughly cooked, turning halfway.
7. Meanwhile, prepare the yogurt sauce: take a medium bowl, add all the ingredients, and whisk until combined.
8. Serve fritters with prepared yogurt sauce.

NUTRITION:

Cal: 94 g
Fat: 2 g
Saturated Fat: 0 g
Carbs: 14 g
Fiber: 3 g
Protein: 4 g
Sugar: 2 g

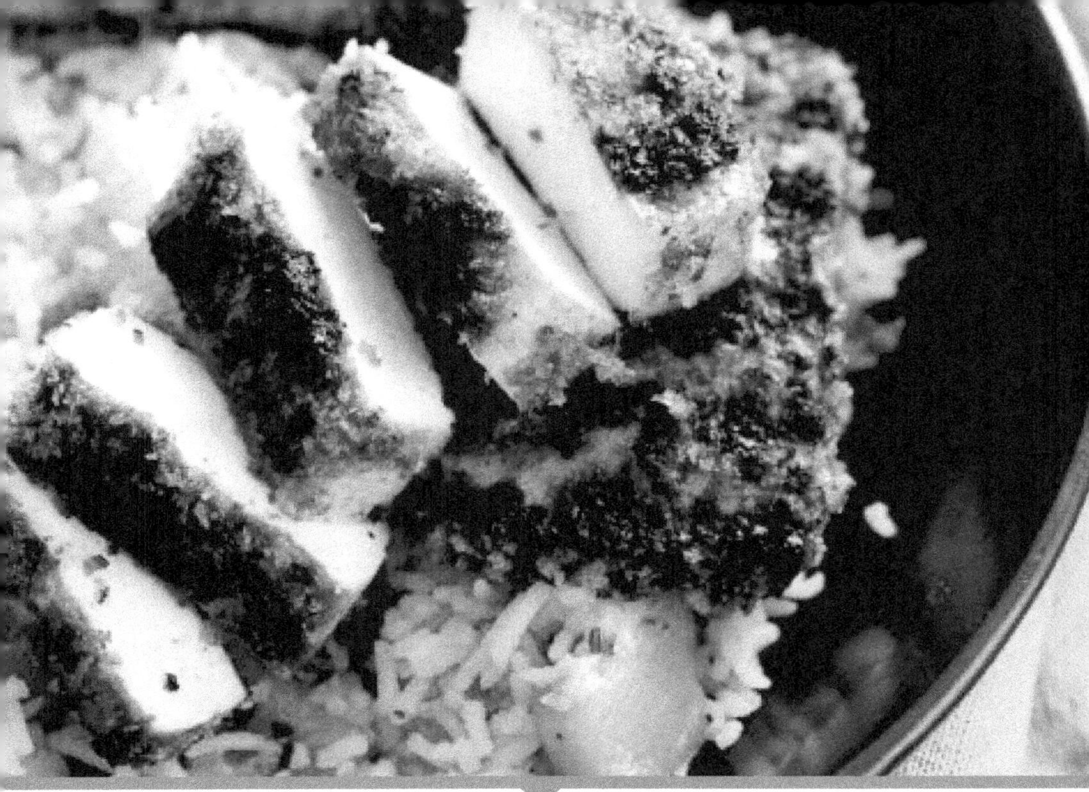

4. BREADED TOFU STEAKS

Preparation Time: 10 Minutes

Cooking Time: 12 Minutes

Servings: 4

INGREDIENTS:

- 3 cups (750 grams) tofu, extra-firm, pressed
- 4 tablespoons tomato paste
- 2 ½ tablespoons minced garlic
- 1 cup (236 grams) panko breadcrumbs and more as needed
- ½ teaspoon ground black pepper
- 2 tablespoon maple syrup
- 2 tablespoons Dijon mustard
- 2 tablespoon soy sauce

- ➢ 4 tablespoons olive oil
- ➢ 2 tablespoon water
- ➢ BBQ sauce for serving

DIRECTIONS:

1. Prepare the tofu steaks: pat dry tofu and then cut them into four slices.
2. Prepare the sauce: take a medium bowl, add garlic, black pepper, maple syrup, mustard, tomato paste, soy sauce, and water; stir until combined.
3. Take a shallow dish and place breadcrumbs on it.
4. Working on one tofu steak at a time, first coat it with prepared sauce, dredge it with breadcrumbs until it is evenly coated, and place it on a plate.
5. Repeat with the remaining tofu slices.
6. Take a frying pan, place it over medium heat, and pour oil in it; when hot, place a tofu steak inside and cook for 4 to 6 minutes per side until golden brown and cooked.
7. Transfer tofu steak to a plate and repeat with the remaining tofu steaks.
8. Serve tofu steaks with the BBQ sauce.

NUTRITION:

Cal: 419.4 g

Fat: 23.9 g

Saturated Fat: 3.9 g

Carbs: 33.3 g

Fiber: 4.3 g

Protein: 22.8 g

Sugar: 3 g

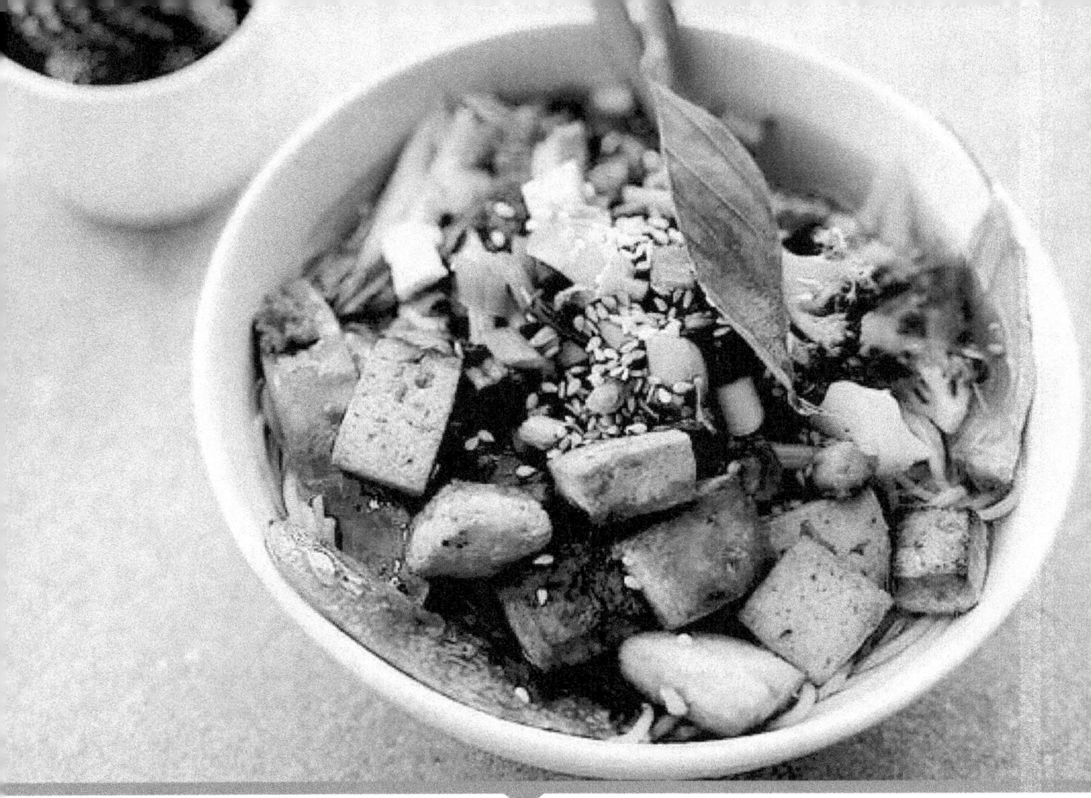

5.   THAI TOFU AND QUINOA BOWLS

Preparation Time: 15 Minutes

Cooking Time: 20 Minutes

Servings: 4

INGREDIENTS:

- ¾ cup (177 grams) quinoa, cooked
- 1 cup (236 grams) frozen edamame, thawed
- 12 ounces (175 grams) tofu, extra-firm, pressed
- 2 medium carrots, grated
- 1 green onion, sliced
- ½ teaspoon minced garlic
- 2 teaspoons grated ginger
- ½ cup chopped cilantro

- ½ teaspoon red chili flakes
- 1 tablespoon soy sauce
- 2 teaspoons agave syrup
- 2 tablespoons lime juice
- 2 tablespoons peanut butter
- 1 tablespoon water
- 4 teaspoons sesame seeds, toasted

DIRECTIONS:

1. Switch on the oven and set it to 400°F, and let it preheat.
2. Prepare the tofu: cut tofu into ¾-inch cubes.
3. Take a large baking sheet, line it with foil, spread tofu pieces on it, and bake until golden brown, stirring halfway.
4. Prepare the drizzle: take a small bowl, place garlic, ginger, chili flakes, soy sauce, agave syrup, butter, lime, and water in it, then whisk until combined.
5. After tofu gets cooked, let it cool for 10 minutes and transfer it into a large bowl.
6. Add carrot, green onions, cilantro, cabbage, and edamame, drizzle with the prepared dressing and sprinkle with sesame seeds.
7. Mix quinoa with salad and serve.

NUTRITION:

Cal: 330 g
Fat: 13 g
Saturated Fat: 3 g
Carbs: 36 g
Fiber: 7 g
Protein: 19 g
Sugar: 10 g

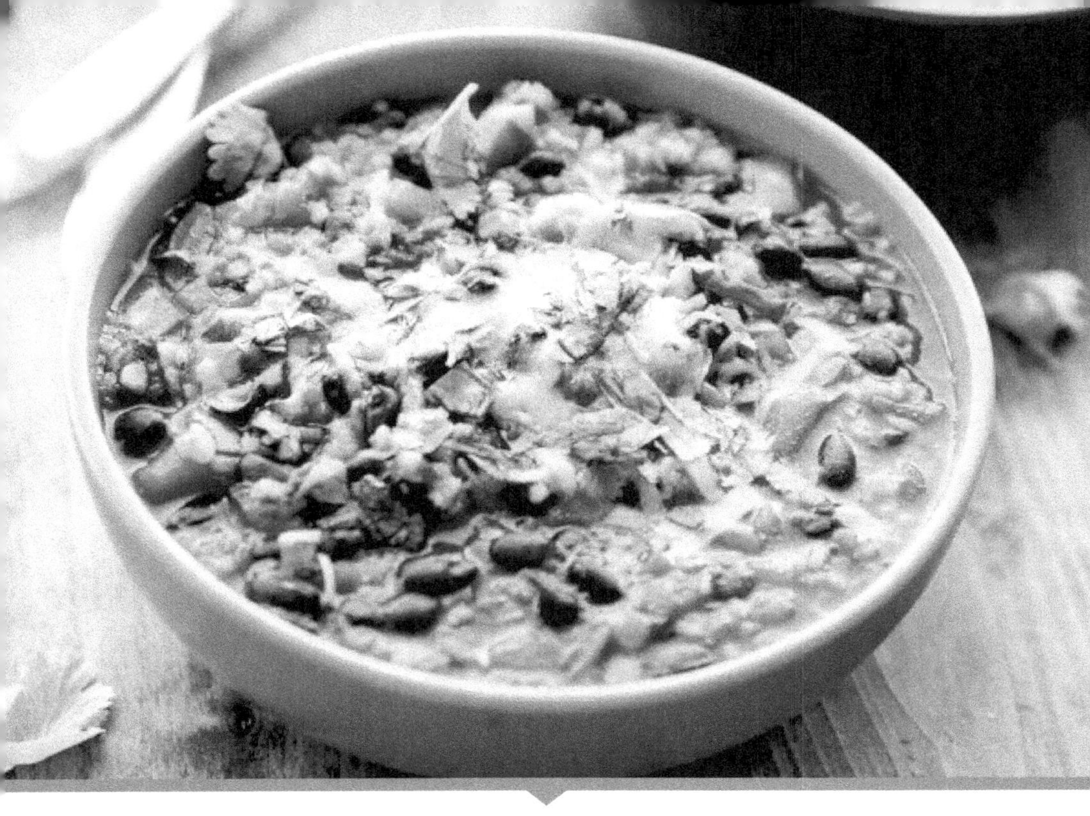

6. BLACK BEAN AND BULGUR CHILI

Preparation Time: 10 Minutes

Cooking Time: 20 Minutes

Servings: 4

INGREDIENTS:

- ¾ cup (177 grams) bulgur wheat, ground
- 30 ounces (850 grams) cooked black beans
- 1 medium red bell pepper, cored, diced
- 1 red onion, peeled, chopped
- 1 medium green bell pepper, cored, diced
- 1 chipotle pepper in adobo sauce, deseeded, diced
- 1 teaspoon minced garlic
- 1 teaspoon smoked paprika

- 1/8 teaspoon sea salt
- 1 teaspoon dried oregano
- 1 teaspoon ground cumin
- 3 cups (710 ml) vegetable broth
- 1 tablespoon olive oil
- 1 lime, juiced
- 1 ¼ cups (295 grams) enchilada sauce

For Topping:

- ½ cup (118 grams) chopped cilantro

DIRECTIONS:

1. Place the large pot over medium-low heat and add oil; when hot, add onion and garlic, season with salt, and cook until softened.
2. Add bell peppers, continue cooking for 5 minutes until tender, add remaining ingredients and stir until mixed.
3. Bring it to a boil, switch heat to a low level and simmer for 10 minutes.
4. Taste to adjust seasoning, then remove the pot from heat, cover it with lid and let it stand for 10 minutes.
5. Distribute chili among bowls, top with cilantro, and serve.

NUTRITION:

Cal: 387 g
Fat: 6.5 g
Saturated Fat: 1.2 g
Carbs: 67.5 g
Fiber: 18.6 g
Protein: 19.8 g
Sugar: 6 g

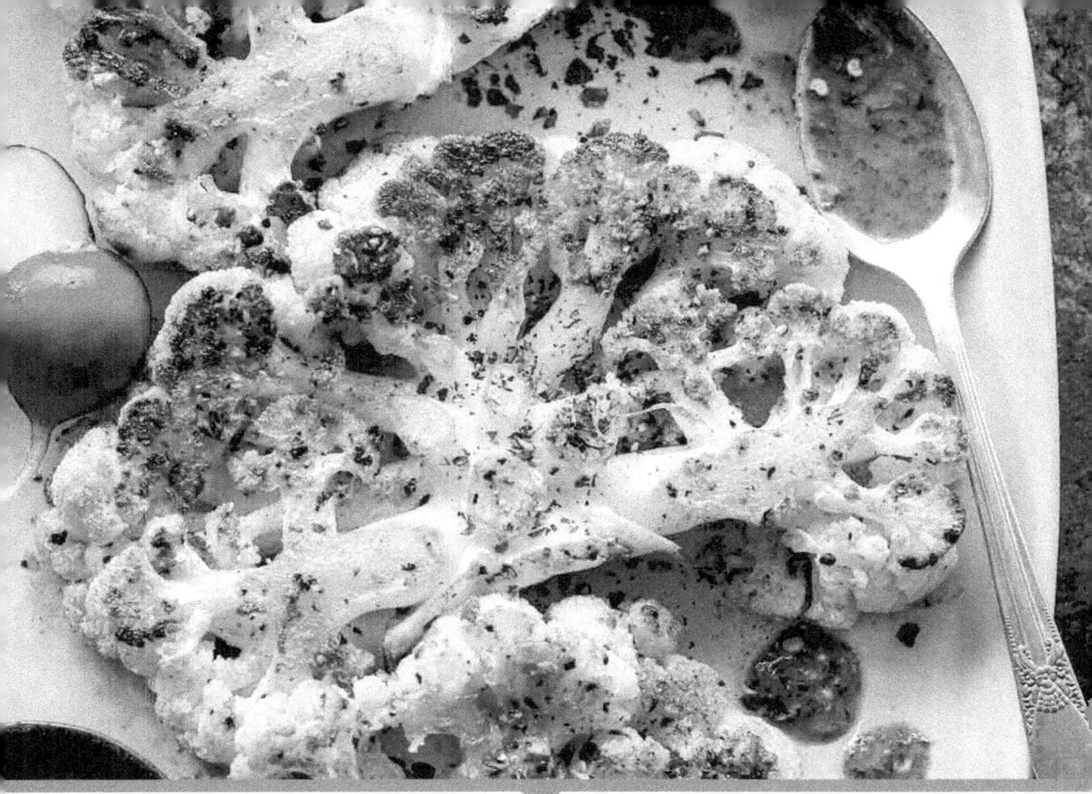

7.   CAULIFLOWER STEAKS

Preparation Time: 10 Minutes

Cooking Time: 30 Minutes

Servings: 3

INGREDIENTS:

- 2 medium heads of cauliflower
- 1 teaspoon garlic powder
- ½ teaspoon ground black pepper
- 1 teaspoon salt
- 1 teaspoon coriander
- 1 teaspoon paprika
- 2 tablespoons olive oil

For Serving:

- ➢ 1 cup (236 grams) hummus

▌ DIRECTIONS:

1. Switch on the oven and set it to 425° F, and let it preheat.
2. Cut each cauliflower head into three slices, brush them with oil on both sides and sprinkle with garlic powder, black pepper, salt, coriander, and paprika.
3. Take a large baking sheet, line it with aluminum foil, arrange cauliflower steaks on it and then bake for 45 minutes until tender and golden brown.
4. Serve straight away.

▌ NUTRITION:

Cal: 149 g
Fat: 9 g
Saturated Fat: 1 g
Carbs: 14 g
Fiber: 7 g
Protein: 5 g
Sugar: 3 g

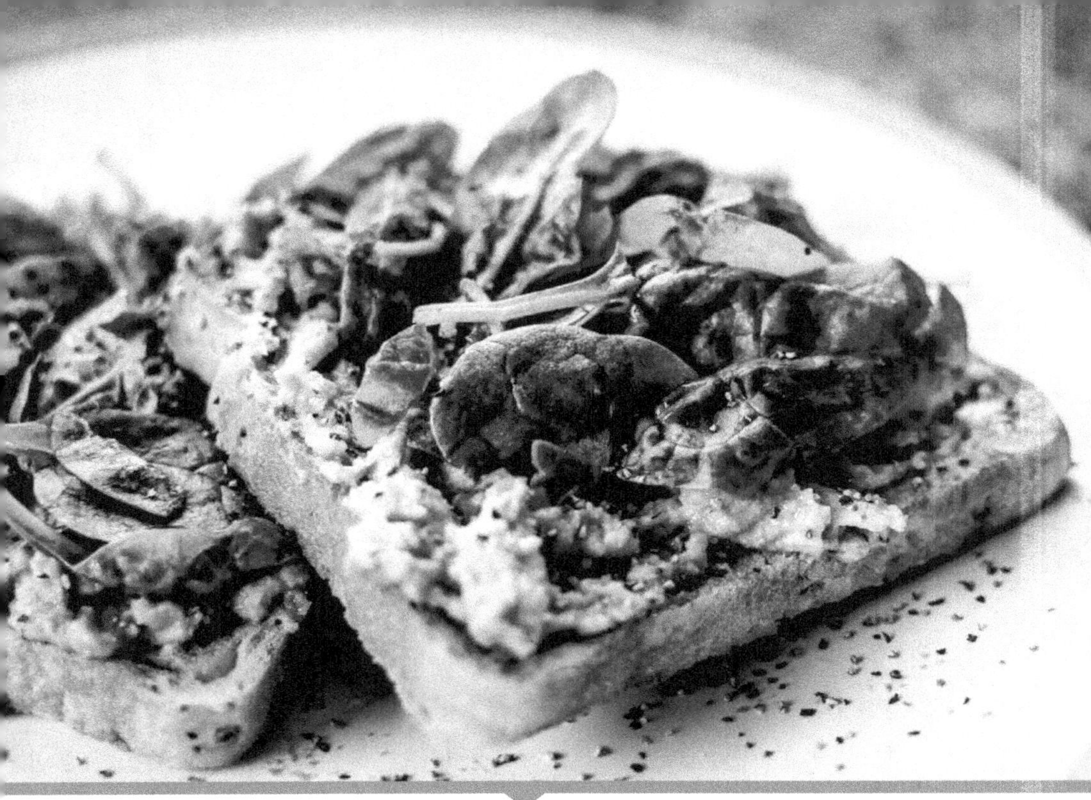

8. AVOCADO AND HUMMUS SANDWICH

Preparation Time: 5 Minutes

Cooking Time: 0 Minutes

Servings: 1

INGREDIENTS:

- 2 slices of whole-wheat bread sliced
- 4 slices of tomato
- 1 lettuce leaf
- ½ avocado, sliced
- 2 tablespoons cilantro leaves
- 2 teaspoons hot sauce
- 3 tablespoon hummuses

DIRECTIONS:

1. Take a slice of bread, spread hummus on its one side, then top with avocado slices and drizzle with hot sauce.
2. Scatter tomato slice on top of avocado slices, then top with lettuce and cilantro and cover with the other slice of bread.
3. Serve straight away.

NUTRITION:

Cal: 302 g
Fat: 5.7 g
Saturated Fat: 1.1 g
Carbs: 49.8 g
Fiber: 12 g
Protein: 12.8 g
Sugar: 7.8 g

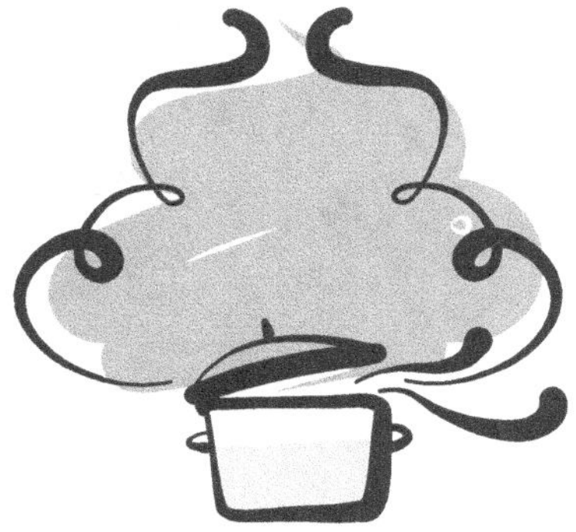

SECOND COURSES

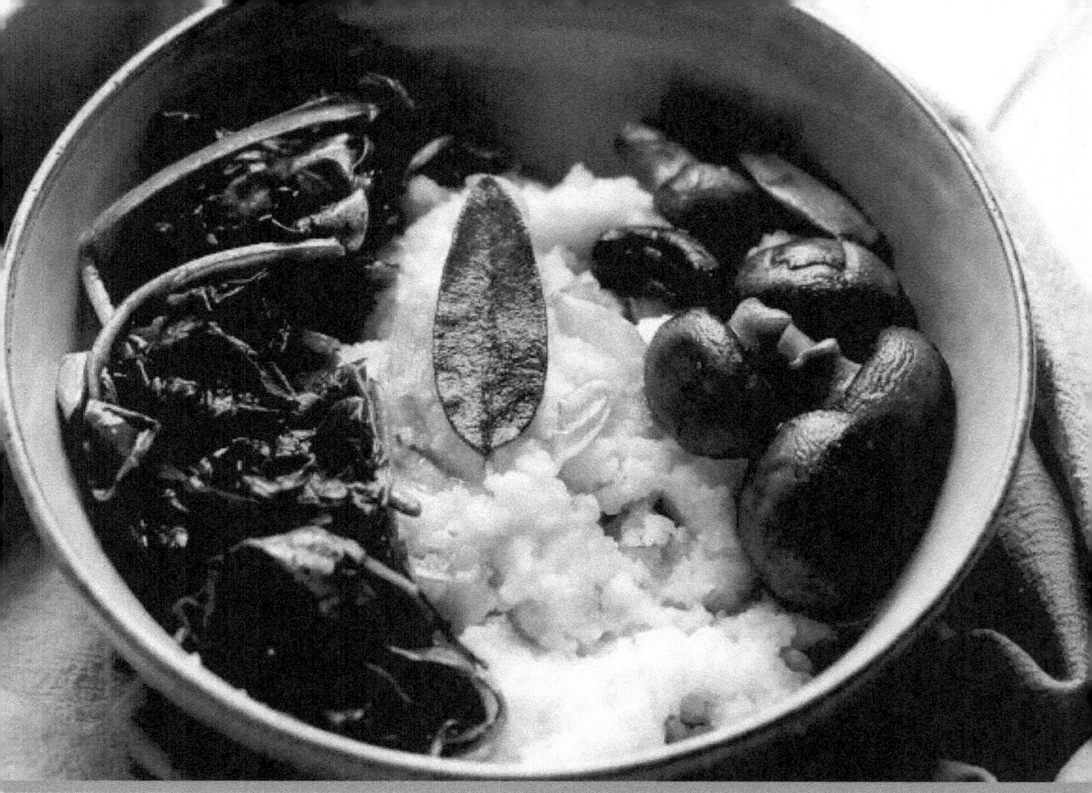

1. CAULIFLOWER MASH WITH SQUASH, MUSHROOMS AND SAGE

Preparation Time: 10 Minutes

Cooking Time: 35 Minutes

Servings: 4

INGREDIENTS:

- 2 tablespoons avocado oil
- ½ white onion, finely chopped
- 2 cups thinly sliced white mushrooms (approximately 5 mushrooms)
- Pinch sea salt
- 4 garlic cloves, minced

- ➢ 1 cauliflower head, coarsely chopped
- ➢ 1 butternut squash, peeled, seeded, and chopped
- ➢ 2 cups low-sodium vegetable stock
- ➢ 3 fresh sage sprigs
- ➢ Freshly ground black pepper, for seasoning

DIRECTIONS:

1. Preheat the oven to 425°F.
2. Heat the oil in a large Dutch oven over medium heat.
3. Add the onion, mushrooms, and salt. Sauté for 5 minutes, or until the mushrooms are cooked through.
4. Add the garlic and cook for 1 minute.
5. Add the cauliflower, squash, stock, and sage.
6. Bring to a boil. Cover and let simmer for 20 minutes, or until the squash and cauliflower are soft.
7. Remove the sage, add the pepper, and mash the mixture until you reach your desired consistency.
8. Bake for 5 to 10 minutes, or until the top begins to turn slightly brown, then serve.

NUTRITION:

Calories: 203
Total fat: 7g
Total carbs: 28g
Cholesterol: 0mg
Fiber: 6g
Sugar: 10g
Protein: 6g
Sodium: 138mg

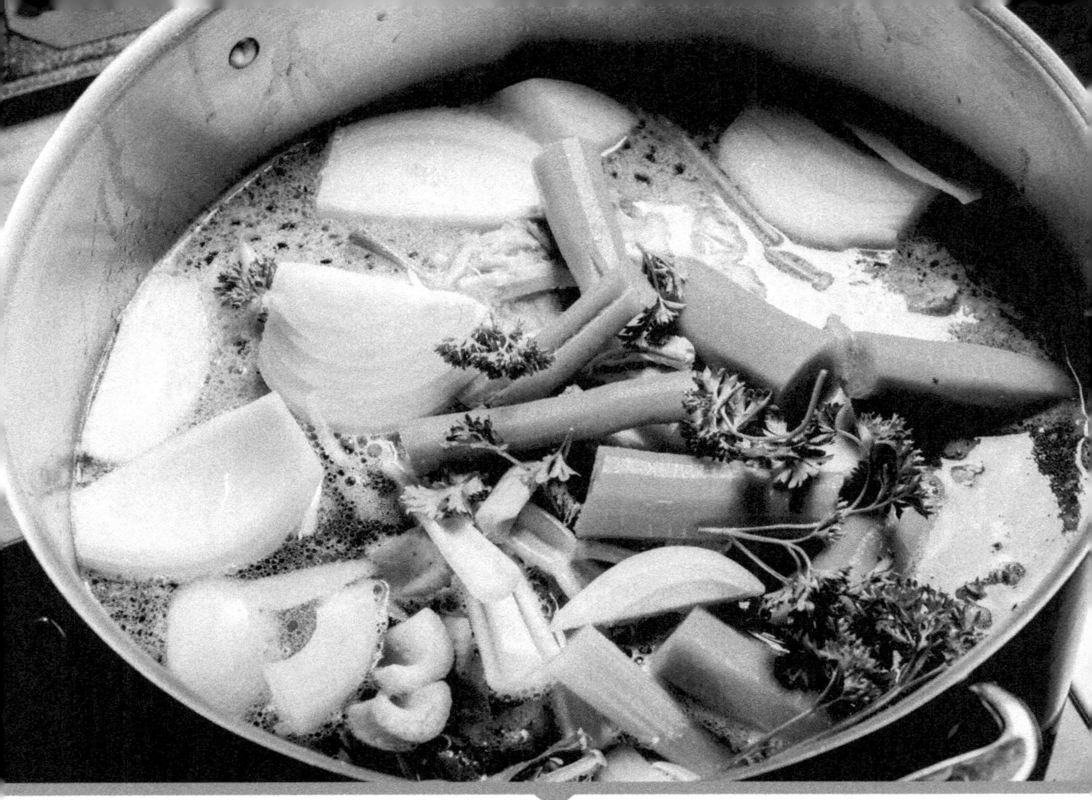

2. BACK-TO-BASICS VEGETABLE STOCK

Preparation Time: 10 Minutes

Cooking Time: 30 Minutes

Servings: 12

INGREDIENTS:

- 1 tablespoon extra-virgin olive oil
- 1 onion, quartered
- 4 large carrots, scrubbed and cut into thirds
- 4 celery stalks, cut into thirds
- ¼ teaspoon sea salt
- 2 garlic cloves
- 4 cups alkaline water
- 1 bunch parsley

DIRECTIONS:

1. Heat the oil in a large Dutch oven over medium heat.
2. Add the onion, carrots, celery, and salt. Sauté for 2 to 3 minutes, stirring frequently, until the onion is translucent.
3. Add the garlic and sauté for 1 minute.
4. Add the water and parsley.
5. Bring to a boil. Cover and let simmer for 30 minutes.
6. Place a fine-mesh strainer over a large glass bowl and strain the liquid. Keep the broth and compost the vegetables.

NUTRITION:

Calories: 27
Total fat: 1g
Total carbs: 4g
Cholesterol: 0mg
Fiber: 2g
Sugar: 2g
Protein: 0g
Sodium: 20mg

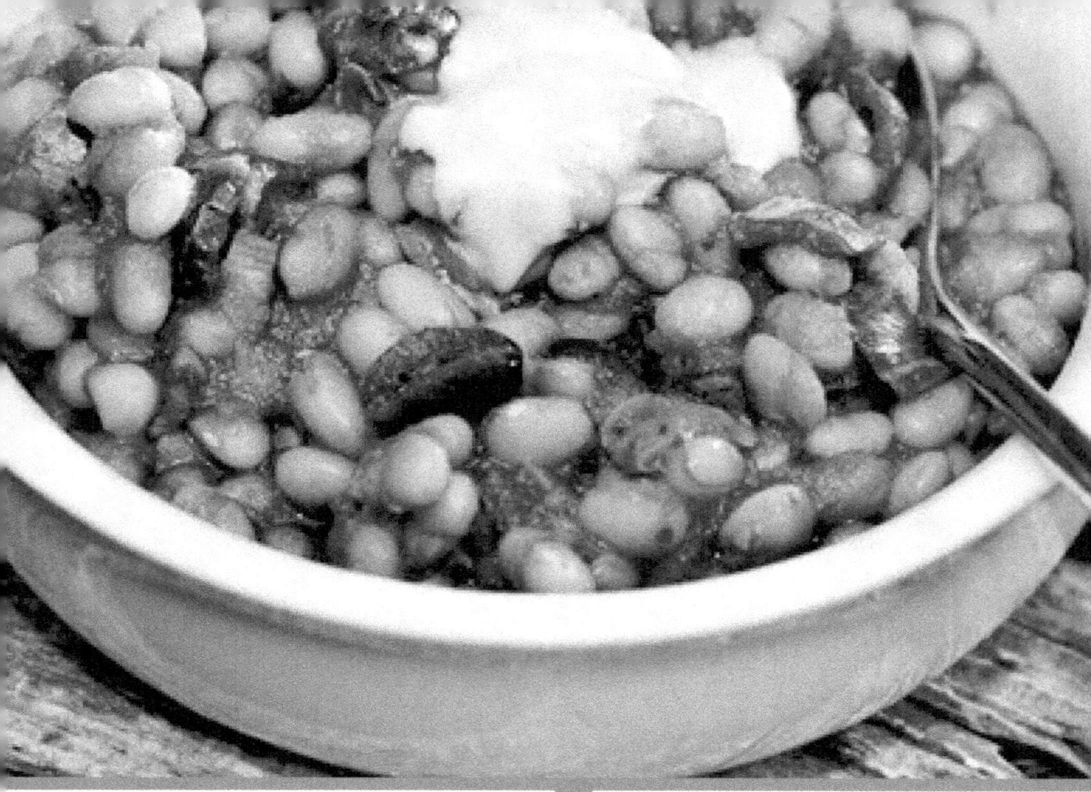

3. CHOCOLATE-MAPLE BAKED BEANS

Preparation Time: 10 Minutes

Cooking Time: 1 Hour and 30 Minutes

Servings: 4

INGREDIENTS:

- 1 sweet onion, finely chopped
- 2 (14-ounce) cans navy beans, drained and rinsed
- ¾ cup blackstrap molasses
- ½ cup pure maple syrup
- 2 tablespoons raw cacao
- 2 tablespoons apple cider vinegar
- Pinch sea salt, for seasoning
- Freshly ground black pepper, for seasoning

DIRECTIONS:

1. Preheat the oven to 325°F.
2. In a large Dutch oven, combine the onion, beans, molasses, syrup, cacao, and vinegar. Season with salt and pepper.
3. Cover and bake for 1½ hours, or until the beans are very tender and the liquid is reduced by half, then serve.

NUTRITION:

Calories: 331
Total fat: 1g
Total carbs: 70g
Cholesterol: 0mg
Fiber: 6g
Sugar: 31g
Protein: 7g
Sodium: 119mg

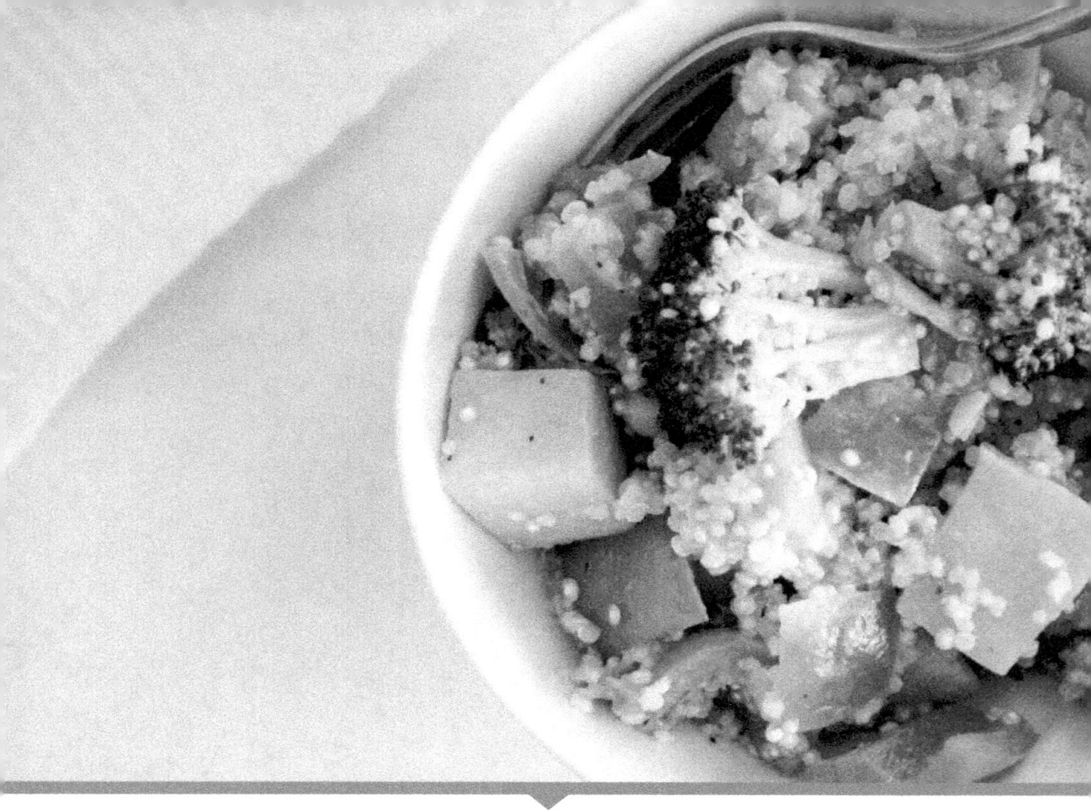

4. GOLDEN MILK QUINOA WITH MAPLE-ROASTED VEGETABLES

Preparation Time: 10 Minutes

Cooking Time: 50 Minutes

Servings: 4

INGREDIENTS:

- ½ red onion, coarsely chopped
- 2 cups broccoli, coarsely chopped
- ½ yam, coarsely chopped
- 1 red bell pepper, coarsely chopped
- 1 teaspoon pure maple syrup
- Pinch sea salt

- ➢ 1 cup quinoa
- ➢ 2 cups full-fat canned coconut milk
- ➢ 1 teaspoon turmeric
- ➢ Pinch freshly ground black pepper

DIRECTIONS:

1. Preheat the oven to 375°F.
2. In a large Dutch oven, combine the onion, broccoli, yam, pepper, syrup, and salt.
3. Bake for 20 minutes, uncovered, or until the veggies are slightly roasted.
4. Remove the vegetables from the oven and turn the heat down to 325°F.
5. Add the quinoa, coconut milk, turmeric, and pepper to the Dutch oven. Mix well.
6. Cover and bake for 30 minutes, or until the quinoa is cooked, then serve.

NUTRITION:

Calories: 437
Total fat: 19g
Total carbs: 54g
Cholesterol: 0mg
Fiber: 9g
Sugar: 8g
Protein: 11g
Sodium: 30mg

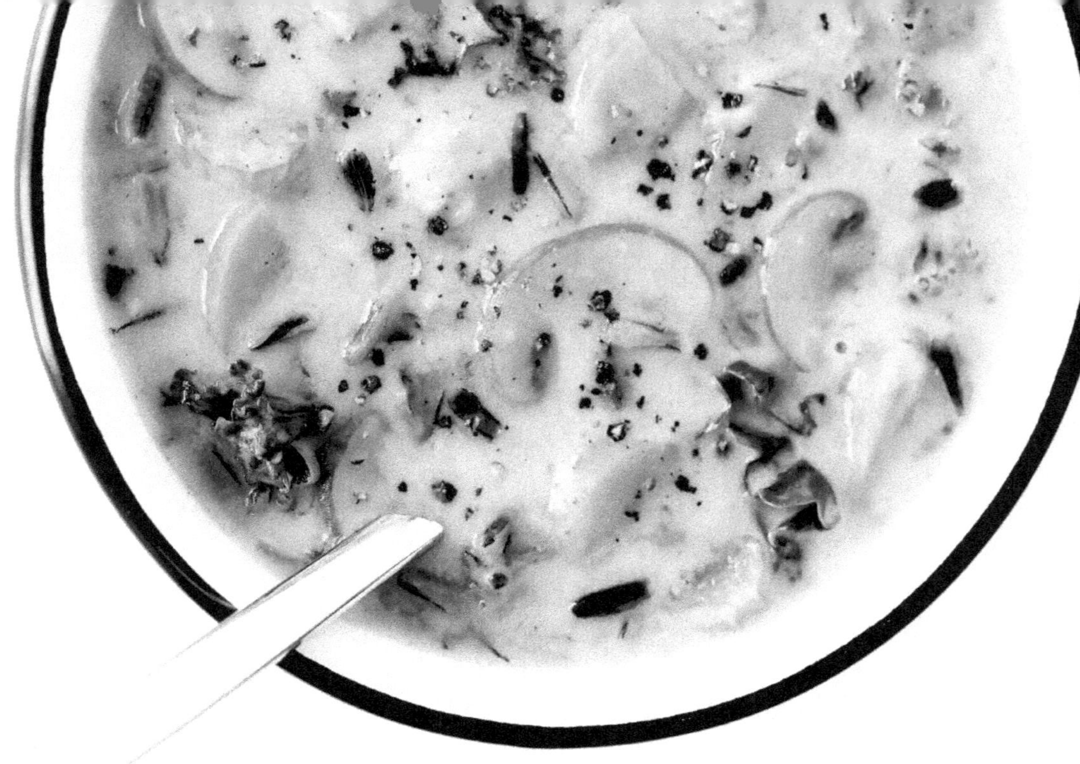

5. COZY AUTUMN VEGETABLE STEW

Preparation Time: 10 Minutes

Cooking Time: 1 Hour and 15 Minutes

Servings: 4

INGREDIENTS:

- 3 tablespoons avocado oil
- 1 white onion, coarsely chopped
- 6 white mushrooms, quartered
- 2 carrots, coarsely chopped
- ½ tablespoon dried thyme
- ½ cup dry red wine
- 1 tablespoon arrowroot powder
- 1 russet potato, coarsely chopped

> 3 cups low-sodium vegetable stock
> Pinch sea salt

DIRECTIONS:

1. Preheat the oven to 325°F.
2. Heat the oil in a large Dutch oven over medium heat.
3. Add the onion, mushrooms, carrots, and thyme. Sauté for 5 minutes, or until the mushrooms begin to soften.
4. Add the wine and arrowroot powder. Stir until it begins to thicken and coat the vegetables, 3 to 4 minutes.
5. Add the potatoes, stock, and sea salt. Bring to a boil for 10 minutes, or until the sauce begins to reduce.
6. Cover and bake for 1 hour, or until the potatoes have softened and the sauce has thickened, then serve.

NUTRITION:

Calories: 207
Total fat: 11g
Total carbs: 22g
Cholesterol: 0mg
Fiber: 3g
Sugar: 5g
Protein: 3g
Sodium: 318mg

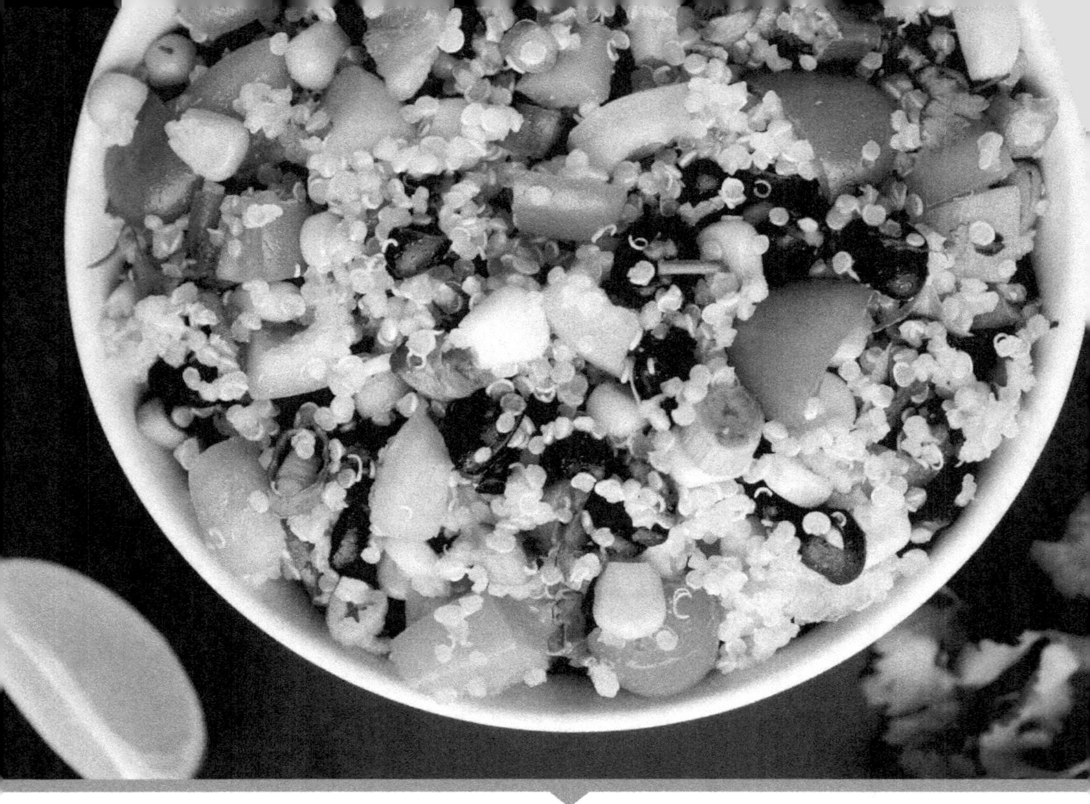

6. MEXICAN CUMIN & LIME QUINOA

Preparation Time: 10 Minutes

Cooking Time: 30 Minutes

Servings: 4

INGREDIENTS:

- 2 tablespoons avocado oil
- ¼ white onion, finely chopped
- Pinch sea salt
- 2 garlic cloves, minced
- 1 cup quinoa
- Juice of ½ lime
- 1 tablespoon ground cumin
- 1 teaspoon chili powder

- ➢ ¼ teaspoon paprika
- ➢ 2 cups low-sodium vegetable stock

DIRECTIONS:

1. Preheat the oven to 325°F.
2. Heat the oil in a large Dutch oven over medium heat.
3. Add the onion and salt. Sauté for 2 to 3 minutes, stirring frequently, until the onion is translucent.
4. Add the garlic, quinoa, lime juice, cumin, chili powder, and paprika. Sauté for 2 minutes.
5. Add the stock and cover with a lid.
6. Bake for 25 minutes, or until the quinoa is cooked, then serve.

NUTRITION:

Calories: 266
Total fat: 8g
Total carbs: 40g
Cholesterol: 0mg
Fiber: 7g
Sugar: 3g
Protein: 9g
Sodium: 70mg

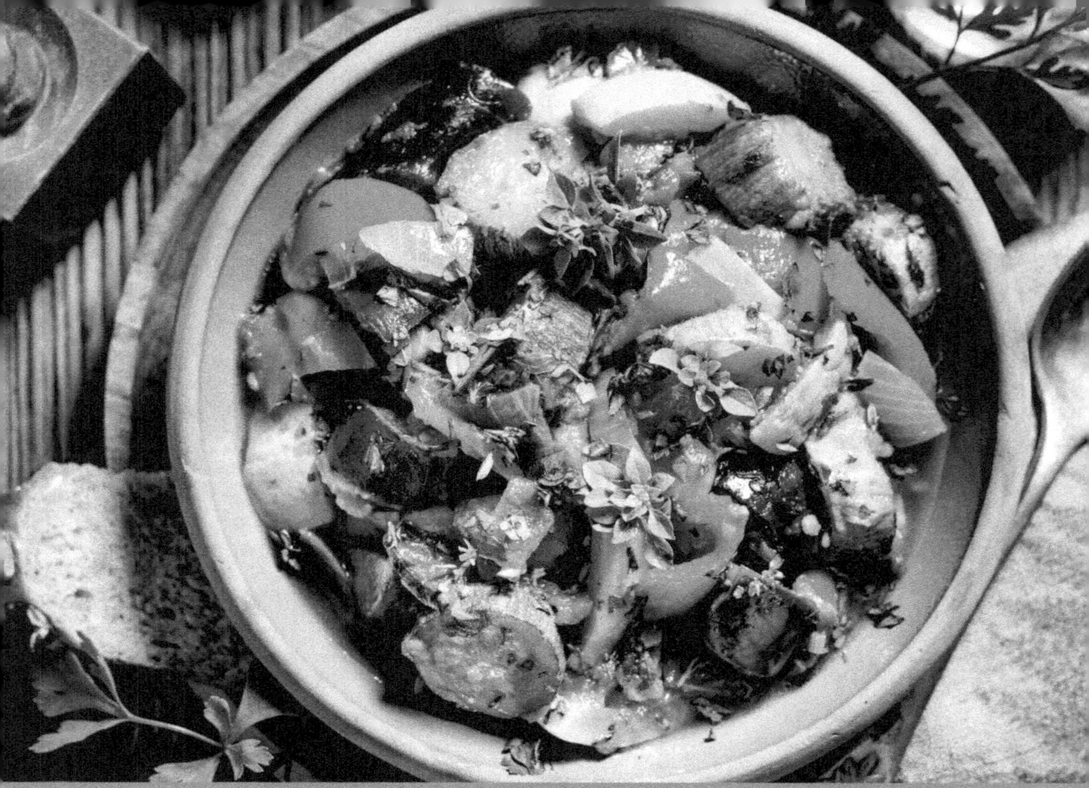

7.   RATATOUILLE

Preparation Time: 10 Minutes

Cooking Time: 50 Minutes

Servings: 4

INGREDIENTS:

- ¼ cup avocado oil
- 1 zucchini, coarsely chopped
- 1 yellow bell pepper, coarsely chopped
- 1 white onion, coarsely chopped
- 8 garlic cloves, coarsely chopped
- Pinch sea salt
- 1 eggplant, coarsely chopped
- 2 (28-ounce) cans low-sodium diced tomatoes, drained

- ➢ ½ cup minced fresh basil
- ➢ 1 teaspoon dried thyme

DIRECTIONS:

1. Preheat the oven to 425°F.
2. In a large Dutch oven, combine the oil, zucchini, pepper, onion, garlic, and salt.
3. Bake, uncovered, for 10 minutes.
4. Remove from the oven and stir in the eggplant. Bake, uncovered, for 20 minutes.
5. Remove from the oven and stir in the diced tomatoes, basil, and thyme.
6. Cook on the stovetop over medium-high heat until it begins to boil.
7. Reduce the heat to low and simmer another 5 to 10 minutes, then serve.

NUTRITION:

Calories: 264
Total fat: 16g
Total carbs: 30g
Cholesterol: 0mg
Fiber: 5g
Sugar: 19g
Protein: 6g
Sodium: 504mg

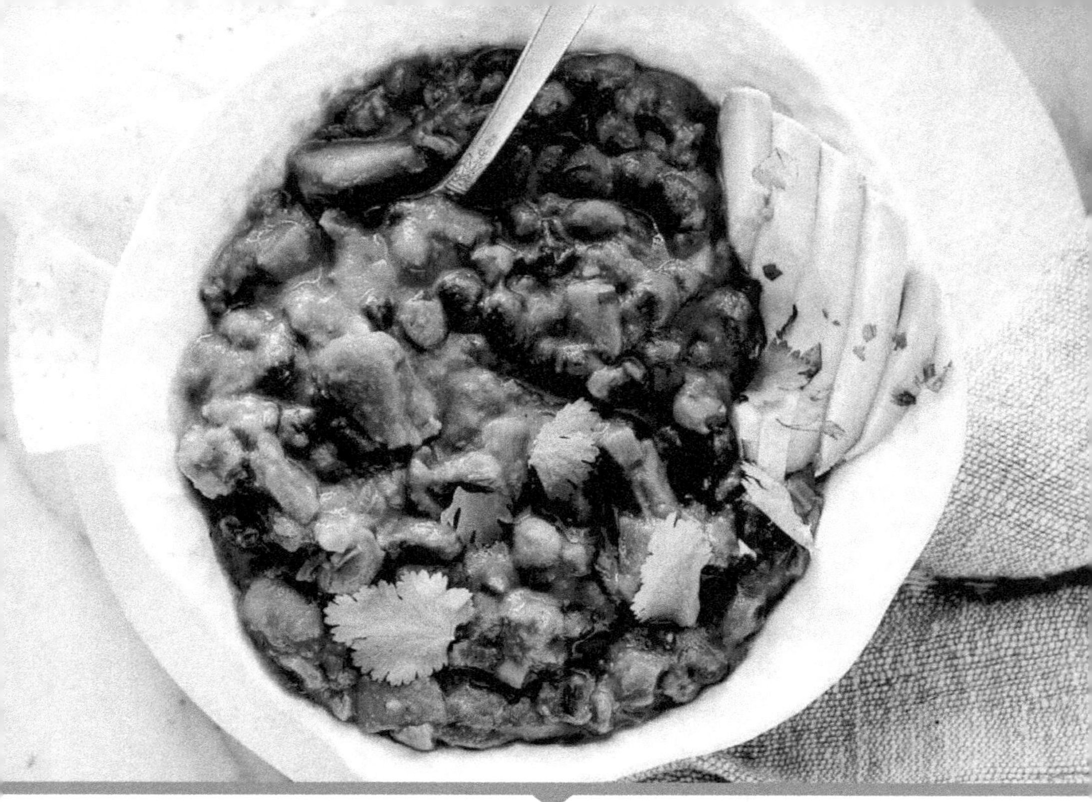

8. SMOKED KIDNEY BEANS
& RED WINE CHILI

Preparation Time: 10 Minutes

Cooking Time: 40 Minutes

Servings: 4

INGREDIENTS:

- 2 tablespoons avocado oil
- ½ red onion, coarsely chopped
- 2 celery stalks, coarsely chopped
- 2 large carrots, coarsely chopped
- 3 garlic cloves, minced
- 1 (19-ounce) can kidney beans, drained and rinsed

- ➢ 1 teaspoon smoked paprika
- ➢ 1 teaspoon chili powder
- ➢ ½ cup dry red wine
- ➢ 1 (28-ounce) can diced tomatoes

DIRECTIONS:

1. Preheat the oven to 325°F.
2. Heat the oil in a large Dutch oven over medium heat.
3. Add the onion, celery, and carrots. Sauté for 2 to 3 minutes, stirring frequently, until the onion is translucent.
4. Add the garlic, kidney beans, and smoked paprika. Mix well and sauté for 2 minutes, stirring frequently.
5. Add the chili powder, red wine, and diced tomatoes. Bring to a boil.
6. Cover and bake for 30 minutes.

NUTRITION:

Calories: 247
Total fat: 9g
Total carbs: 31g
Cholesterol: 0mg
Fiber: 9g
Sugar: 10g
Protein: 10g
Sodium: 476mg

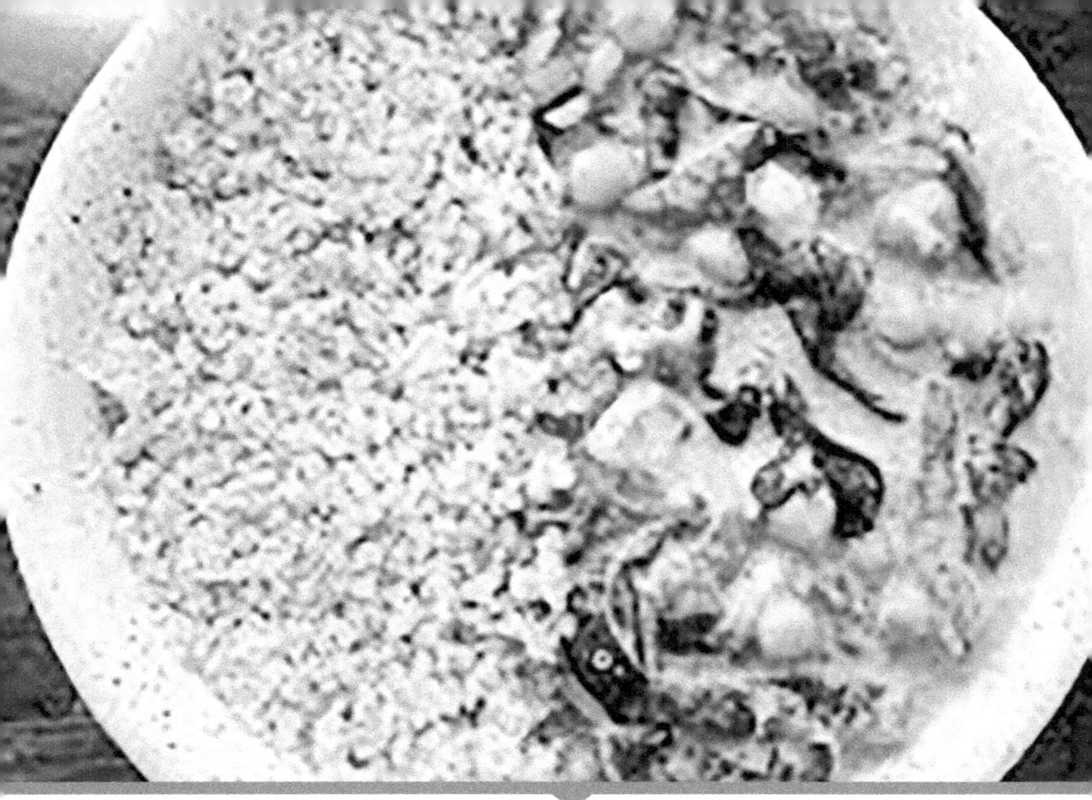

9. SUN-DRIED TOMATO, COCONUT-BRAISED BOK CHOY & NAVY BEANS

Preparation Time: 10 Minutes

Cooking Time: 30 Minutes

Servings: 4

INGREDIENTS:

- 2 tablespoons avocado oil
- 1 white onion, finely chopped
- 6 garlic cloves, minced
- Pinch sea salt
- ½ cup oil-packed sun-dried tomatoes, finely chopped
- 1 (14-ounce) can navy beans, drained and rinsed

- ➢ 4 baby bok choy, thoroughly cleaned and coarsely chopped
- ➢ 2 (14-ounce) cans coconut milk
- ➢ Pinch freshly ground black pepper
- ➢ Juice of 1 lemon

DIRECTIONS:

1. Preheat the oven to 325°F.
2. Heat the oil in a large Dutch oven over medium-low heat.
3. Add the onion, garlic, and salt. Sauté for 5 minutes, stirring frequently, until the onion is translucent.
4. Add the sun-dried tomatoes and sauté for 1 minute.
5. Increase the heat to high and stir in the navy beans. Cook, stirring frequently, for 2 minutes.
6. Add the bok choy and stir until it becomes bright in color, about 1 minute.
7. Stir in the coconut milk and pepper until well mixed.
8. Cover and bake for 20 minutes.
9. Add the lemon juice before serving.

NUTRITION:

Calories: 539
Total fat: 27g
Total carbs: 75g
Cholesterol: 0mg
Fiber: 28g
Sugar: 8g
Protein: 26g
Sodium: 66mg

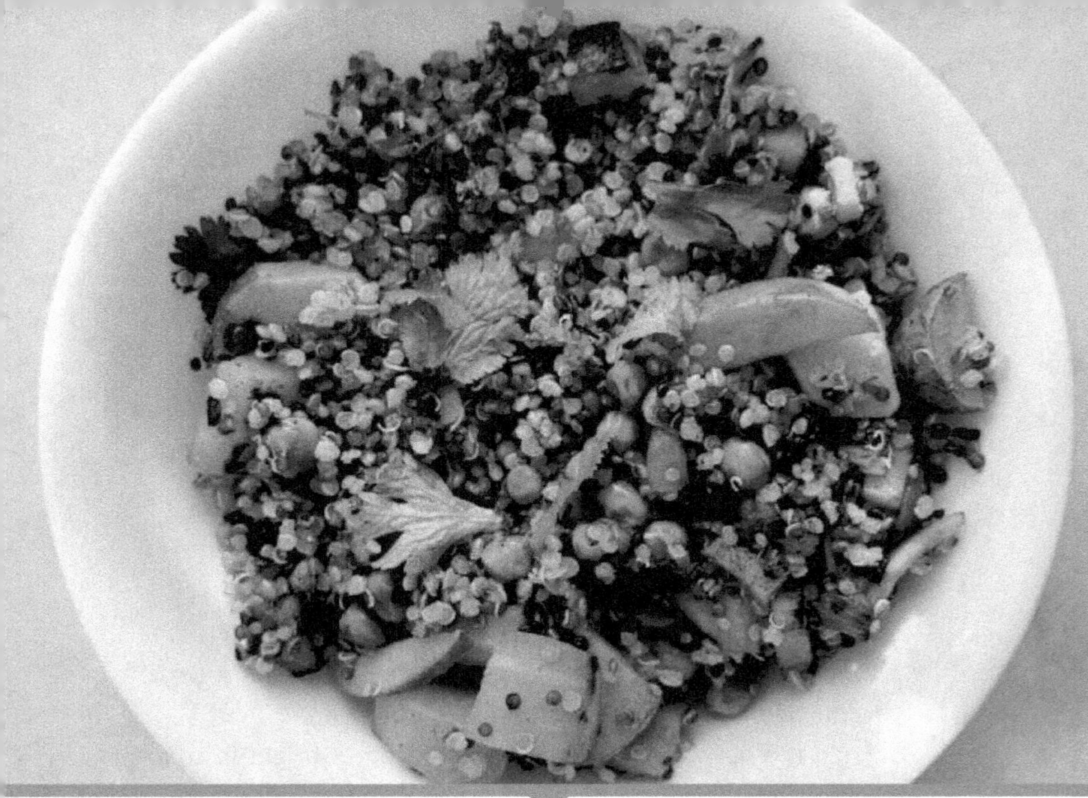

10. QUINOA MASALA

Preparation Time: 10 Minutes

Cooking Time: 45 Minutes

Servings: 4

INGREDIENTS:

- ½ white onion, chopped
- Pinch sea salt, plus more for seasoning
- 1 red bell pepper, chopped
- ½ jalapeño pepper, seeded and finely chopped
- 2 tablespoons fresh ginger, peeled and grated
- 1 (19-ounce) can black beans, drained and rinsed
- 1 tablespoon garam masala powder
- 1 cup quinoa

- ➤ 2 cups low-sodium vegetable stock
- ➤ Juice of ½ lemon

DIRECTIONS:

1. Preheat the oven to 375° F.
2. In a large Dutch oven, sauté the onion and salt for 2 to 3 minutes, stirring frequently, until the onion is translucent.
3. Add the pepper, jalapeño, ginger, black beans, and garam masala. Sauté for 2 minutes.
4. Add the quinoa and stock. Cover and bake for 40 minutes.
5. Add the lemon juice and fluff with a fork before serving.
6. Adjust seasoning with salt and serve.

NUTRITION:

Calories: 503
Total fat: 3g
Total carbs: 103g
Cholesterol: 0mg
Fiber: 25g
Sugar: 7g
Protein: 32g
Sodium: 80mg

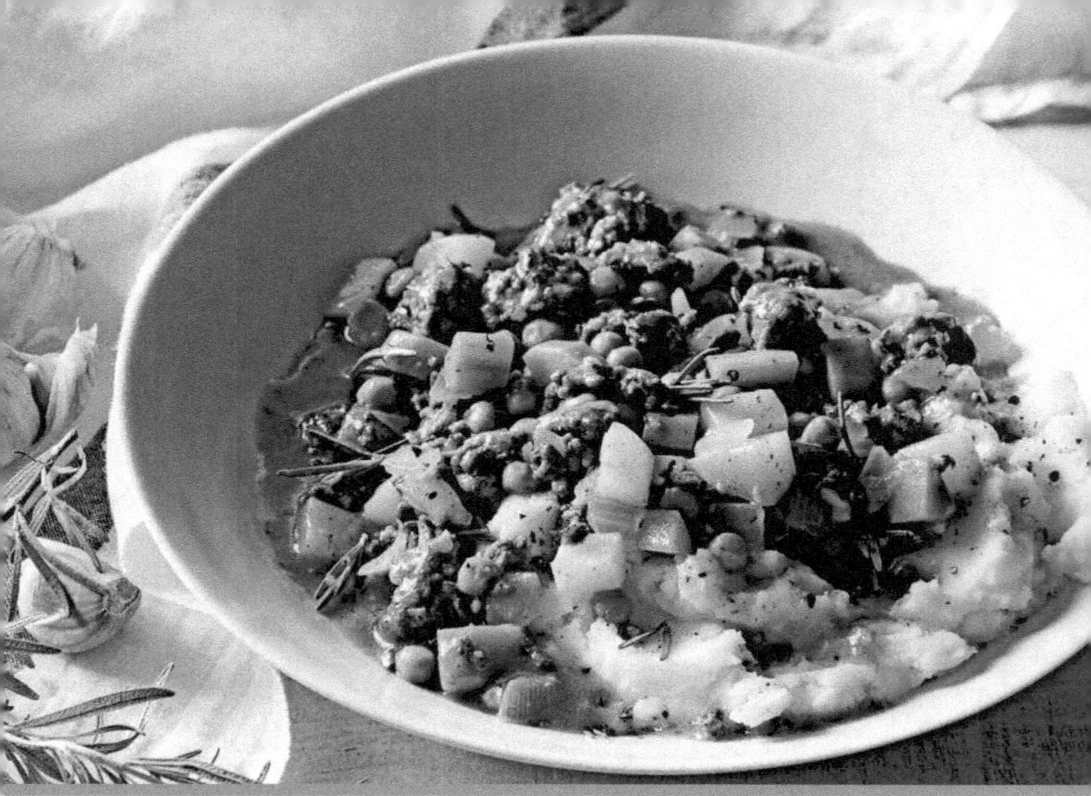

11. UPSIDE-DOWN VEGAN SHEPHERD'S PIE

Preparation Time: 10 Minutes

Cooking Time: 50 Minutes

Servings: 4

INGREDIENTS:

- 2 russet potatoes, peeled and cut into 1-inch chunks
- 6 garlic cloves, minced
- 2 cups low-sodium vegetable stock
- Pinch sea salt, plus more for seasoning
- Pinch freshly ground black pepper
- 1 teaspoon dried thyme

- ➢ 1 cup chopped carrots
- ➢ 1 cup chopped green beans
- ➢ 2 cups finely chopped portobello mushrooms

DIRECTIONS:

1. Preheat the oven to 425°F.
2. In a large Dutch oven, combine the potatoes, garlic, stock, salt, and pepper.
3. Cover and bake for 30 minutes.
4. Remove from the oven and mash the potatoes right in the Dutch oven. Add the thyme and mix well. Spread the potatoes evenly at the bottom of the Dutch oven.
5. Top with the carrots, green beans, and mushrooms. Sprinkle with a pinch of sea salt.
6. Cover and bake for 20 minutes, then serve.

NUTRITION:

Calories: 122
Total fat: 0g
Total carbs: 28g
Cholesterol: 0mg
Fiber: 4g
Sugar: 5g
Protein: 5g
Sodium: 99mg

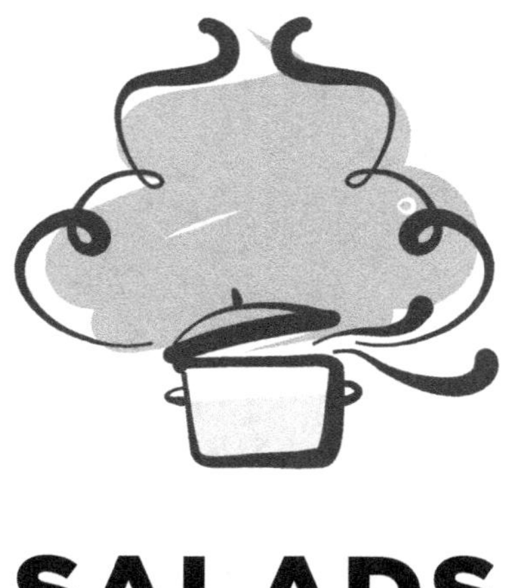

SALADS

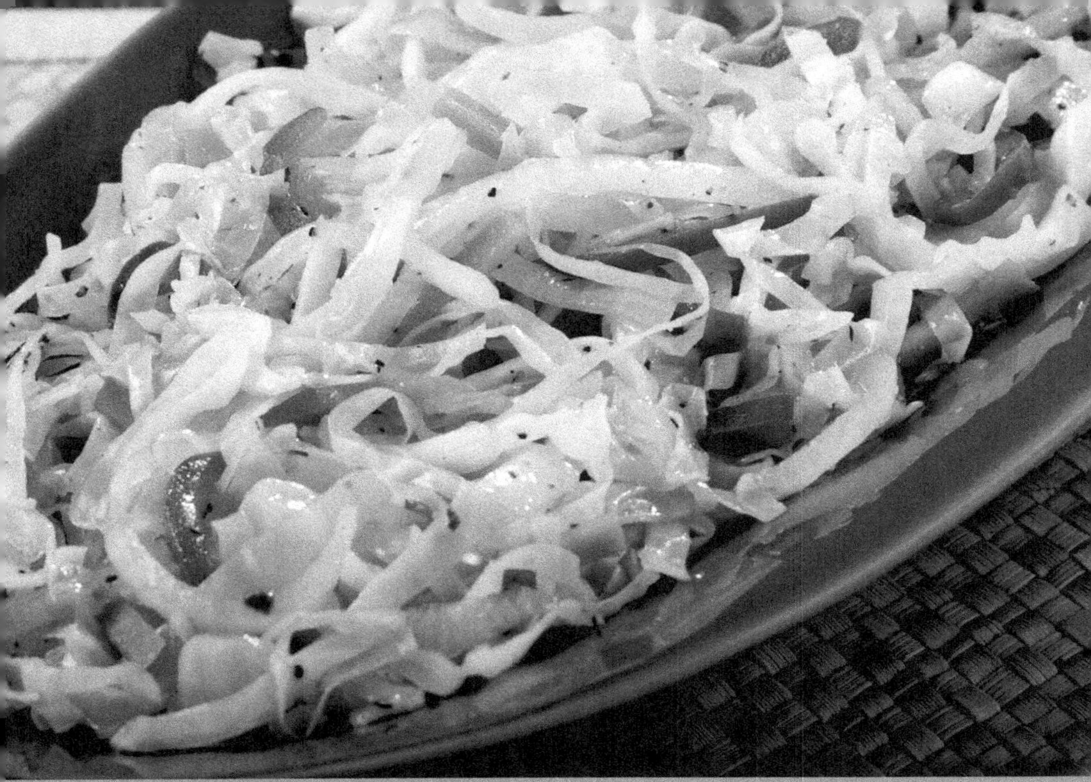

1.   HOT CABBAGE QUARTET SALAD

Preparation Time: 5 Minutes

Cooking Time: 15 Minutes

Servings: 4

INGREDIENTS:

- 3 tablespoons extra-virgin olive oil
- ½ yellow onion, rinsed and finely chopped
- 8 ounces cabbage, rinsed and shredded
- 8 ounces broccoli, rinsed and cut into medium-size pieces
- 8 ounces bok choy, rinsed and chopped
- 8 ounces Brussels sprouts, rinsed and halved
- 1 tablespoon rinsed and finely chopped celery
- 1½ teaspoons fresh thyme leaves, rinsed and finely chopped

- ➢ 1 teaspoon garlic powder
- ➢ ½ teaspoon Himalayan pink salt, plus more as needed
- ➢ ½ teaspoon freshly ground black pepper
- ➢ ¾ cup filtered water
- ➢ 1 tablespoon freshly squeezed lemon juice

DIRECTIONS:

1. Coat the interior of an electric pressure cooker with the olive oil. In the pot, combine the onion, cabbage, broccoli, bok choy, Brussels sprouts, celery, thyme, garlic powder, salt, and pepper. Stir well.
2. Add the water, and stir again.
3. Lock the lid into place, select Manual and High Pressure, and cook for 6 minutes.
4. Once the beep hums, rapid release the pressure by choosing Cancel and winding the steam regulator to the Venting position. Cautiously remove the cover and transfer the vegetables to a serving bowl.
5. Taste and season with salt, as needed. Drizzle with the lemon juice and serve.

NUTRITION:

Calories: 144.7
Total Fat: 10.49g
Total Carbohydrates: 9.86g
Fiber: 4.1g
Sugar: 4g
Protein: 3.71g

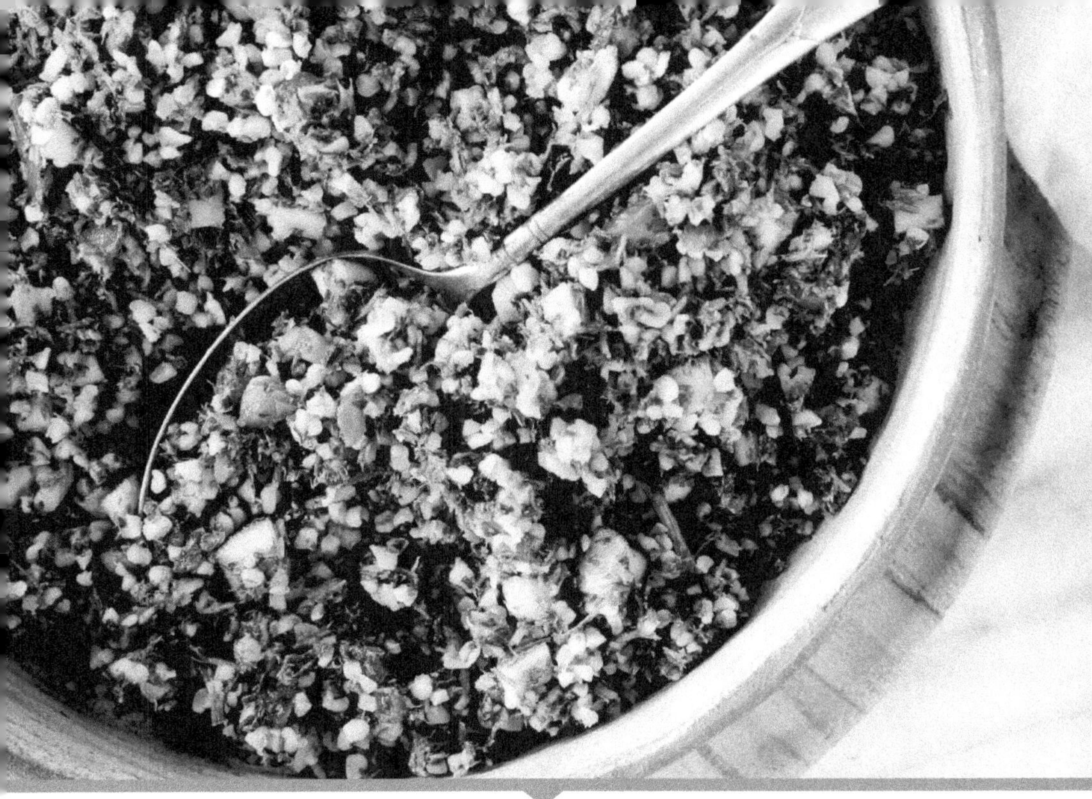

2. TABBOULEH SALAD

Preparation Time: 20 Minutes

Cooking Time: 15 Minutes

Servings: 4

INGREDIENTS:

- 2 cups filtered water
- 1 cup millet, rinsed
- ⅓ cup extra-virgin olive oil
- Juice of 1 lemon
- 1 large garlic clove, crushed
- 1½ teaspoons Himalayan pink salt, divided
- 2 large tomatoes, rinsed and finely diced
- 3 scallions, white parts only, rinsed and thinly sliced

- ½ English cucumber, rinsed and finely diced
- ¾ cup fresh mint, rinsed and finely chopped
- 1½ cups fresh parsley, rinsed and finely chopped

DIRECTIONS:

1. In a small saucepan over high heat, bring the water to boil. Add the millet and turn the heat to low. Cover the pan and cook for 15 minutes.
2. Remove the pan from the heat and mash the millet with a fork. Let cool with the lid off for 15 minutes. The texture should be firm but not crunchy or mushy.
3. Meanwhile, in a small bowl, whisk the olive oil, lemon juice, garlic, and ½ teaspoon of salt. Let sit.
4. In a large bowl, combine the tomatoes, scallions, cucumber, mint, and parsley.
5. Add the cooled millet. Pour the dressing over and mix well. Taste and season with the remaining 1 teaspoon of salt, as needed.

NUTRITION:

Calories: 360
Total Fat: 20g
Total Carbohydrates: 44g
Fiber: 8g
Sugar: 3g
Protein: 8g

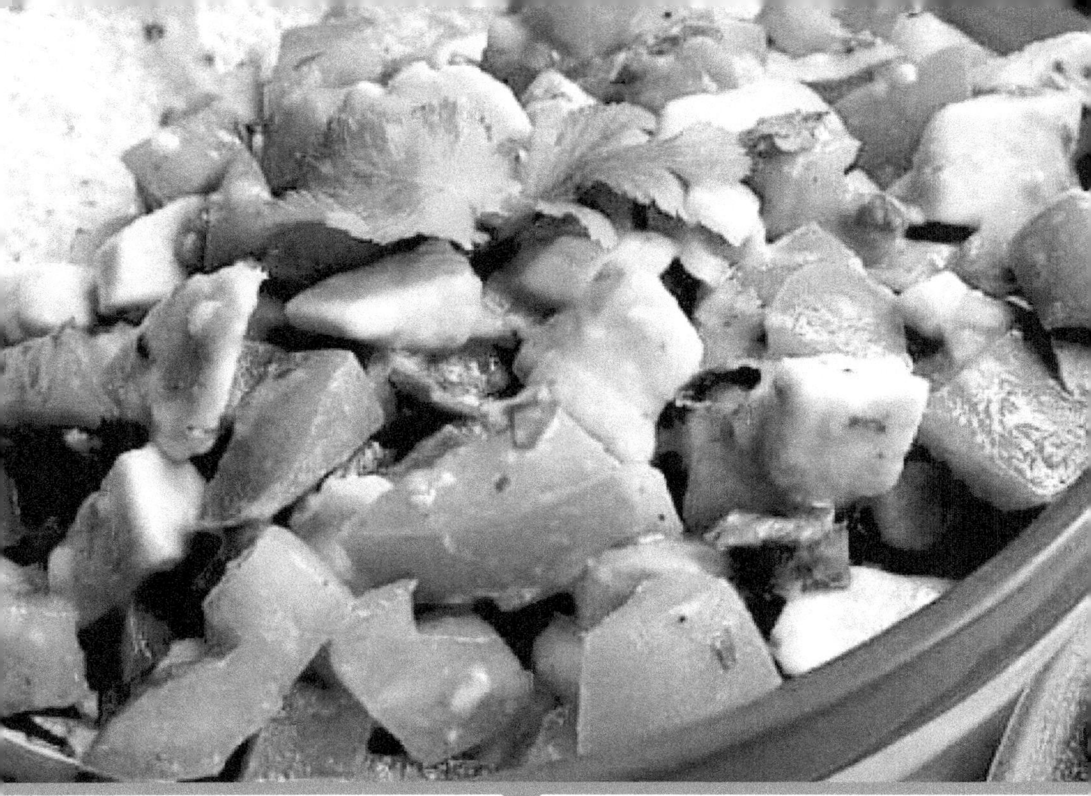

3. GUACAMOLE SALAD

Preparation Time: 10 Minutes

Cooking Time: 0 Minutes

Servings: 2

INGREDIENTS:

- 2 avocados, halved and pitted
- ½ cup diced red onion
- ½ cup fresh cilantro, rinsed and chopped
- Juice of ½ lime
- ½ teaspoon onion powder
- ½ teaspoon ground cayenne
- ½ teaspoon Himalayan pink salt
- 1 tomato, rinsed and diced

▍ DIRECTIONS:

1. Scoop the avocado flesh into a medium bowl.
2. Add the red onion, cilantro, lime juice, onion powder, cayenne, and salt. Mash everything until smooth.
3. Add the tomato, mix well, and serve.

▍ NUTRITION:

Calories: 450
Total Fat: 40g
Total Carbohydrates: 27g
Fiber: 16g
Sugar: 5g
Protein: 5g

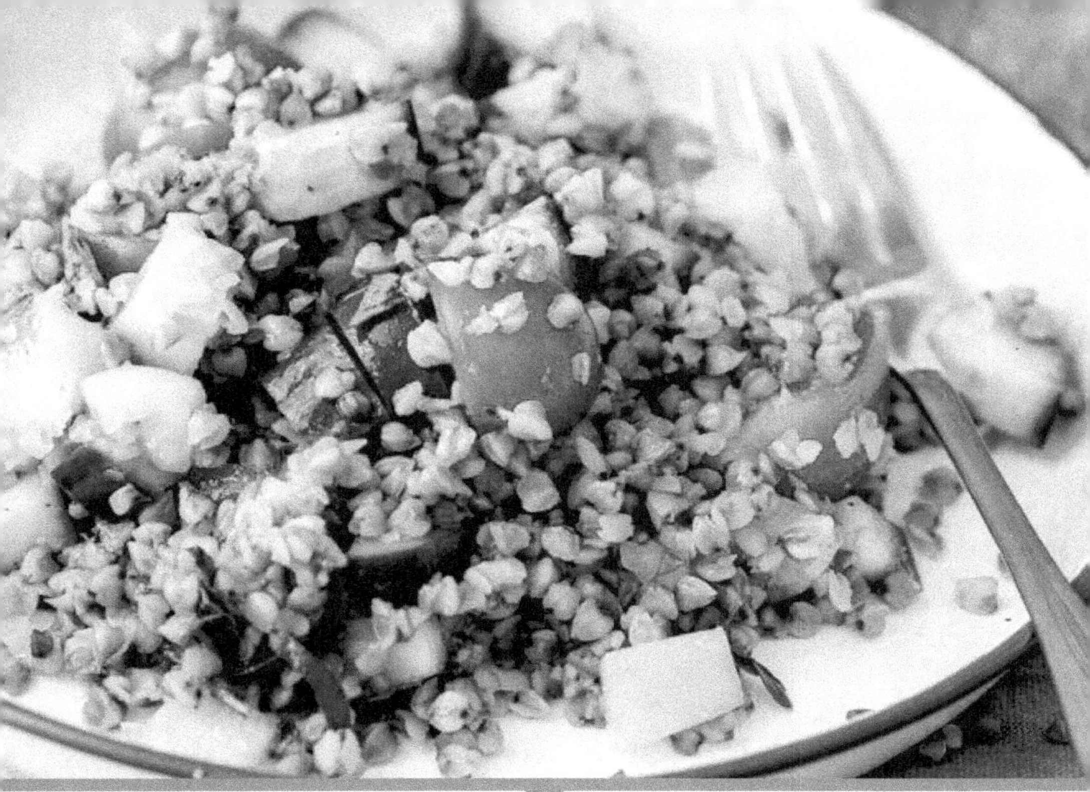

4.   BUCKWHEAT SALAD

Preparation Time: 10 Minutes

Cooking Time: 15 Minutes

Servings: 2

INGREDIENTS:

- 1 cup raw buckwheat, rinsed
- 2 cups water
- 2 handfuls fresh baby spinach leaves, rinsed
- Handful fresh basil leaves, rinsed
- 2 scallions, white parts only, rinsed and chopped
- Zest of 1 lemon
- Juice of ½ lemon
- ½ red onion, finely chopped

- ➢ Himalayan pink salt
- ➢ Freshly ground black pepper
- ➢ ¼ cup extra-virgin olive oil
- ➢ 1 red chile, rinsed and thinly sliced
- ➢ 2 tablespoons mixed sprouts, rinsed
- ➢ 1 ripe avocado, peeled, pitted, and sliced
- ➢ 1½ ounces feta cheese (optional)

DIRECTIONS:

1. In a medium saucepan, combine the buckwheat and water, and bring to a boil over high heat. Reduce the heat to simmer and cook for 15 minutes, or until soft. Remove from the heat and let cool.
2. Meanwhile, in a food processor, combine the baby spinach, basil, scallions, lemon zest, and lemon juice, and process for 30 seconds.
3. Stir the herb mixture into the cooled buckwheat.
4. Add the red onion and season with salt and pepper.
5. Arrange the buckwheat on a platter. Drizzle with the olive oil and scatter on the chopped chile and sprouts. Top with the sliced avocado, crumble the feta over top (if using), and serve.

NUTRITION:

Calories: 685
Total Fat: 54g
Total Carbohydrates: 43g
Fiber: 16g
Sugar: 5g
Protein: 14g

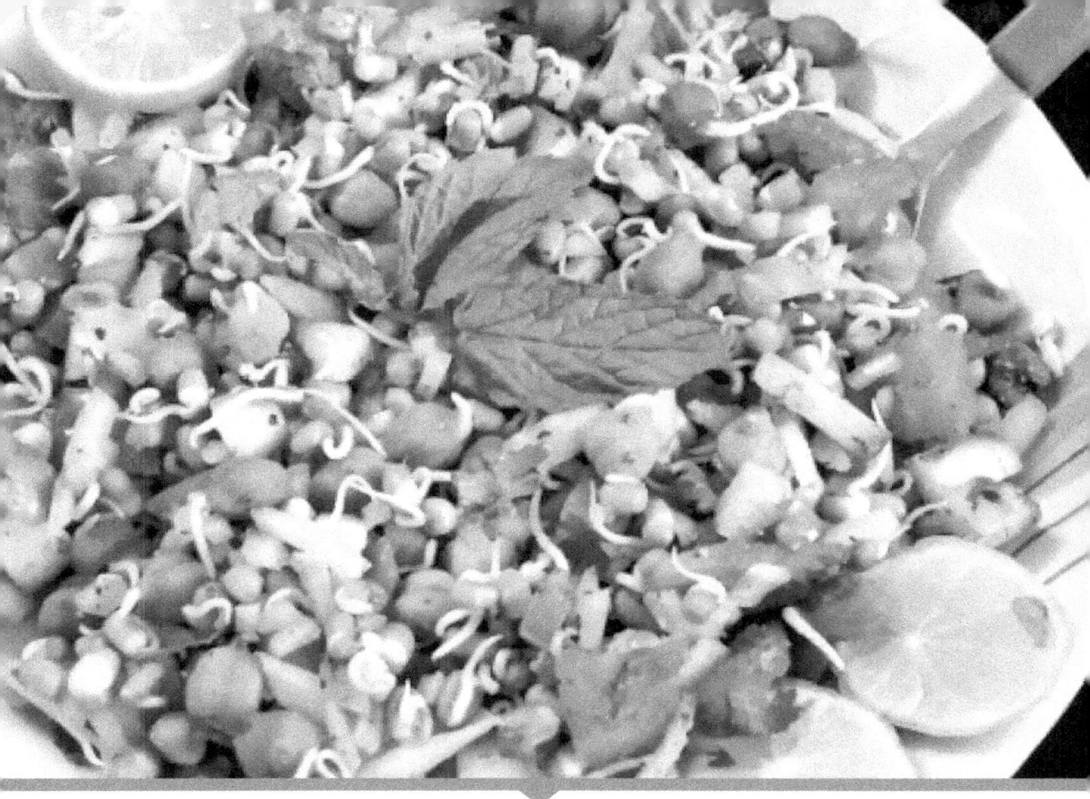

5. MIXED SPROUTS SALAD

Preparation Time: 10 Minutes

Cooking Time: 0 Minutes

Servings: 2

INGREDIENTS:

- 1 to 2 tablespoons coconut oil
- Juice of 1 lemon
- Handful fresh chives, rinsed and chopped
- Handful fresh dill, rinsed and chopped
- Handful fresh parsley, rinsed and chopped
- ½ teaspoon Himalayan pink salt
- ½ teaspoon freshly ground black pepper
- 1 scallion, rinsed and chopped

- ➢ 1 cucumber, rinsed and chopped
- ➢ ½ cup mixed sprouts of choice (alfalfa, radish, broccoli, mung bean, cress, etc.), rinsed

DIRECTIONS:

1. In a blender, combine the coconut oil, lemon juice, chives, dill, parsley, salt, and pepper, and blend until mainly smooth. Transfer to a medium bowl.
2. Stir in the scallion, cucumber, and sprouts to coat, and serve.

NUTRITION:

Calories: 168
Total Fat: 14g
Total Carbohydrates: 12g
Fiber: 1g
Sugar: 4g
Protein: 3g

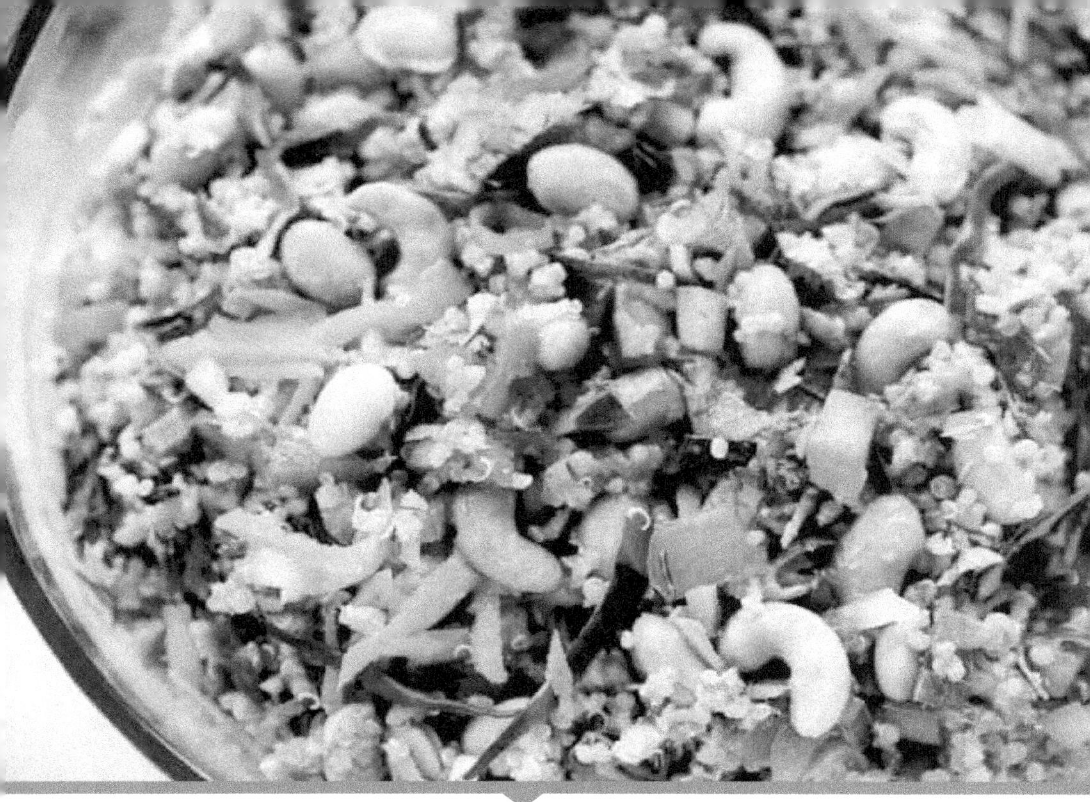

6.   THAI QUINOA SALAD

Preparation Time: 15 Minutes

Cooking Time: 0 Minutes

Servings: 2

INGREDIENTS:

For the dressing

- ⅓ cup filtered water
- ¼ cup tahini
- 1 pitted date
- 1 tablespoon sesame seeds
- 1 tablespoon apple cider vinegar
- 2 teaspoons tamari

- ➢ 1 teaspoon freshly squeezed lemon juice
- ➢ 1 teaspoon toasted sesame oil
- ➢ 1 teaspoon chopped garlic
- ➢ ½ teaspoon Himalayan pink salt

For the salad

- ➢ 1 cup quinoa, rinsed and steamed
- ➢ 1 cup arugula, rinsed and chopped
- ➢ 1 tomato, rinsed and sliced
- ➢ ¼ red onion, rinsed and diced

▍DIRECTIONS:

To make the dressing

1. In a blender, combine the water, tahini, date, sesame seeds, vinegar, tamari, lemon juice, sesame oil, garlic, and salt. Blend on high speed until smooth.

To make the salad

2. In a medium bowl, stir together the quinoa, arugula, tomato, and red onion. Add the dressing, stir well to coat, and serve.

▍NUTRITION:

Calories: 558
Total Fat: 25g
Total Carbohydrates: 69g
Fiber: 10g
Sugar: 4g
Protein: 19g

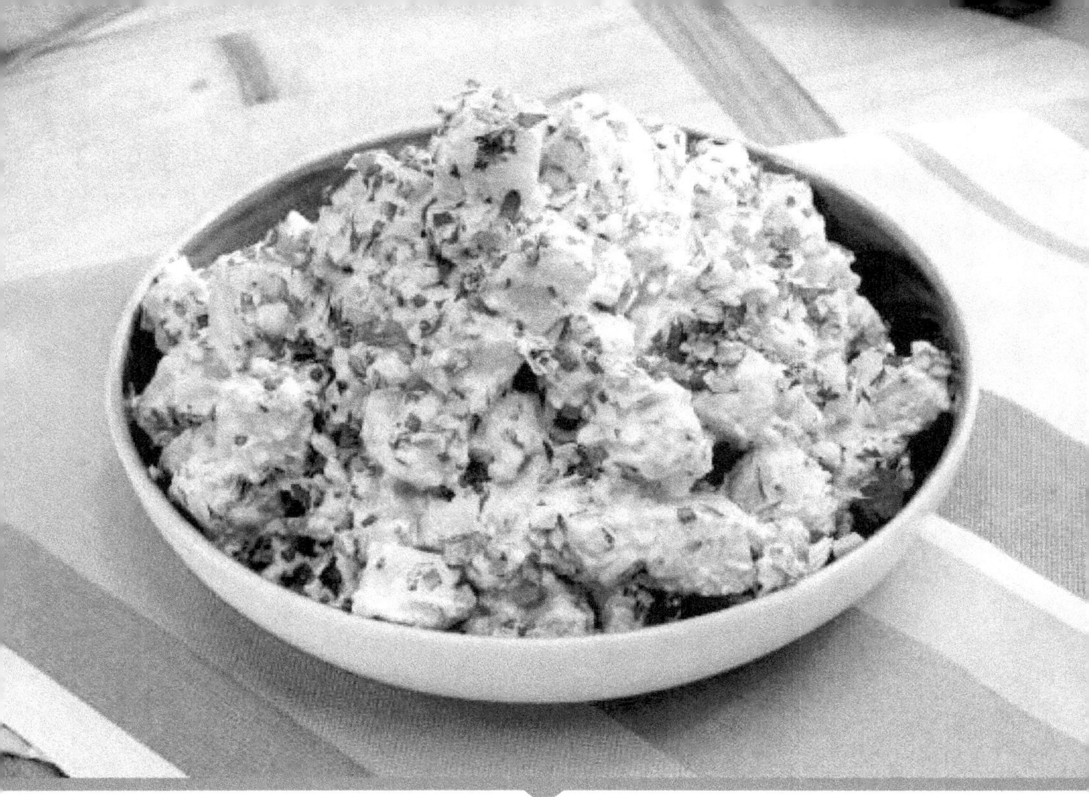

7. SWEET POTATO SALAD

Preparation Time: 15 Minutes

Cooking Time: 5 Minutes

Servings: 2

INGREDIENTS:

For the dressing

- ½ cup sesame oil
- 2 tablespoons coconut oil
- 2 tablespoons light soy sauce
- 1 tablespoon coconut sugar or raw honey
- 1 garlic clove, crushed

For the salad

- ➢ 5½ ounces fresh baby spinach leaves, rinsed
- ➢ 1 red onion, rinsed and finely chopped
- ➢ 1 tomato, rinsed, seeded, and chopped
- ➢ 1 tablespoon coconut oil
- ➢ 1 large sweet potato, scrubbed, peeled, and diced

DIRECTIONS:

To make the dressing

1. In a small bowl, whisk the sesame oil, coconut oil, soy sauce, coconut sugar, and garlic until blended. Set aside.

To make the salad

2. In a large salad bowl, gently toss together the baby spinach, red onion, and tomato. Set aside.
3. In a small skillet over medium heat, heat the coconut oil. Add the sweet potato and cook for 3 to 5 minutes, stirring, until golden brown. Using a slotted spoon, add the sweet potato to the salad and gently stir to combine.
4. Pour the dressing over the salad, gently toss again to coat, and serve.

NUTRITION:

Calories: 550
Total Fat: 52g
Total Carbohydrates: 20g
Fiber: 3g
Sugar: 9g
Protein: 3g

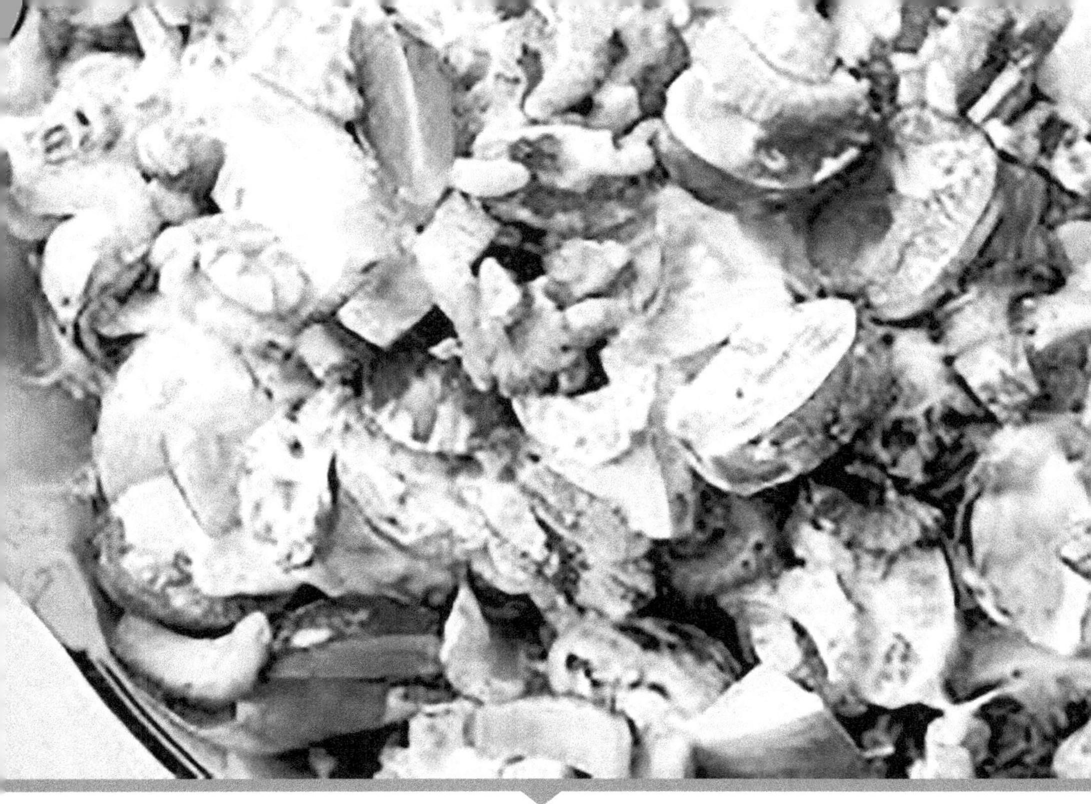

8. WALDORF SALAD

Preparation Time: 15 Minutes

Cooking Time: 0 Minutes

Servings: 2

INGREDIENTS:

For the dressing

- 1 ripe avocado, peeled and pitted
- 1 teaspoon Dijon mustard
- ½ teaspoon Himalayan pink salt
- Freshly ground black pepper
- Juice of ½ lemon

For the salad

- ➢ 2 cups canned chickpeas, rinsed and drained, or cooked, drained, and cooled
- ➢ 1 cup sunflower seeds, soaked in filtered water overnight, drained
- ➢ 2 apples, rinsed, cored, and chopped
- ➢ ½ red onion, rinsed and diced
- ➢ 1 celery stalk, rinsed and diced
- ➢ 1 to 2 teaspoons chopped fresh dill, rinsed

DIRECTIONS:

To make the dressing

1. In a small bowl, using a fork, mash together the avocado, mustard, salt, pepper, and lemon juice. Set aside.

To make the salad

2. In a large bowl, stir together the chickpeas, sunflower seeds, and dressing until well combined.
3. Stir in the apples, red onion, and celery. Top with the fresh dill and serve.

NUTRITION:

Calories: 700
Total Fat: 40g
Total Carbohydrates: 80g
Fiber: 28g
Sugar: 15g
Protein: 28g

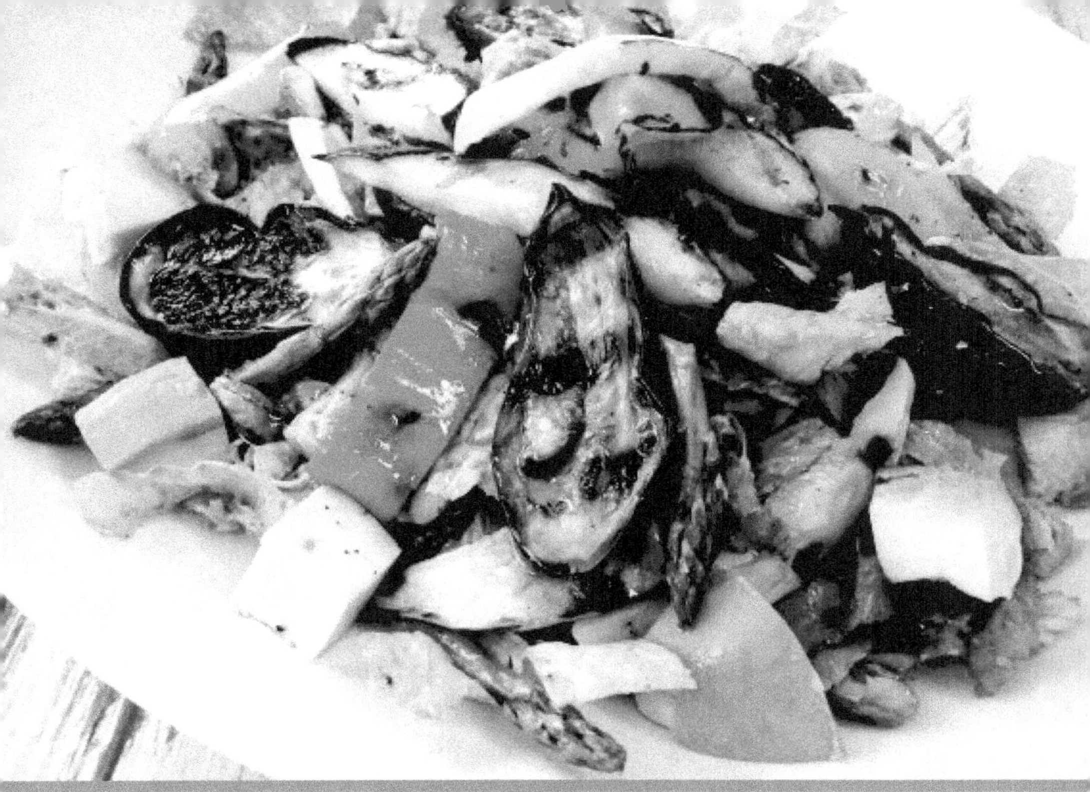

9.   ITALIAN ROASTED VEGETABLE SALAD

Preparation Time: 15 Minutes

Cooking Time: 25 Minutes

Servings: 2

INGREDIENTS:

- 1 cup mushrooms, rinsed and chopped
- 1 zucchini, rinsed and chopped
- 1 red onion, rinsed and sliced
- 1 yellow squash, rinsed and cut into medium chunks
- 1 green bell pepper, rinsed and cut into thin strips
- 1 red bell pepper, rinsed and cut into thin strips
- 3 tablespoons extra-virgin olive oil
- 1½ teaspoons Italian seasoning

> ➤ ½ teaspoon Himalayan pink salt
> ➤ ¼ teaspoon freshly ground black pepper
> ➤ 1 teaspoon dried parsley

DIRECTIONS:

1. Preheat the oven to 425°F. Line a large baking sheet with parchment paper and set aside.
2. In a large bowl, combine the mushrooms, zucchini, red onion, yellow squash, and green and red bell peppers. Drizzle the olive oil over the veggies and stir to mix well.
3. Add the Italian seasoning, salt, pepper, and parsley, and stir well again until fully mixed. Spread the veggies on the prepared baking sheet in a single layer.
4. Roast for 25 minutes, stirring the vegetables halfway through the cooking time, or until tender.

NUTRITION:

Calories: 270
Total Fat: 20g
Total Carbohydrates: 18g
Fiber: 6g
Sugar: 10g
Protein: 5g

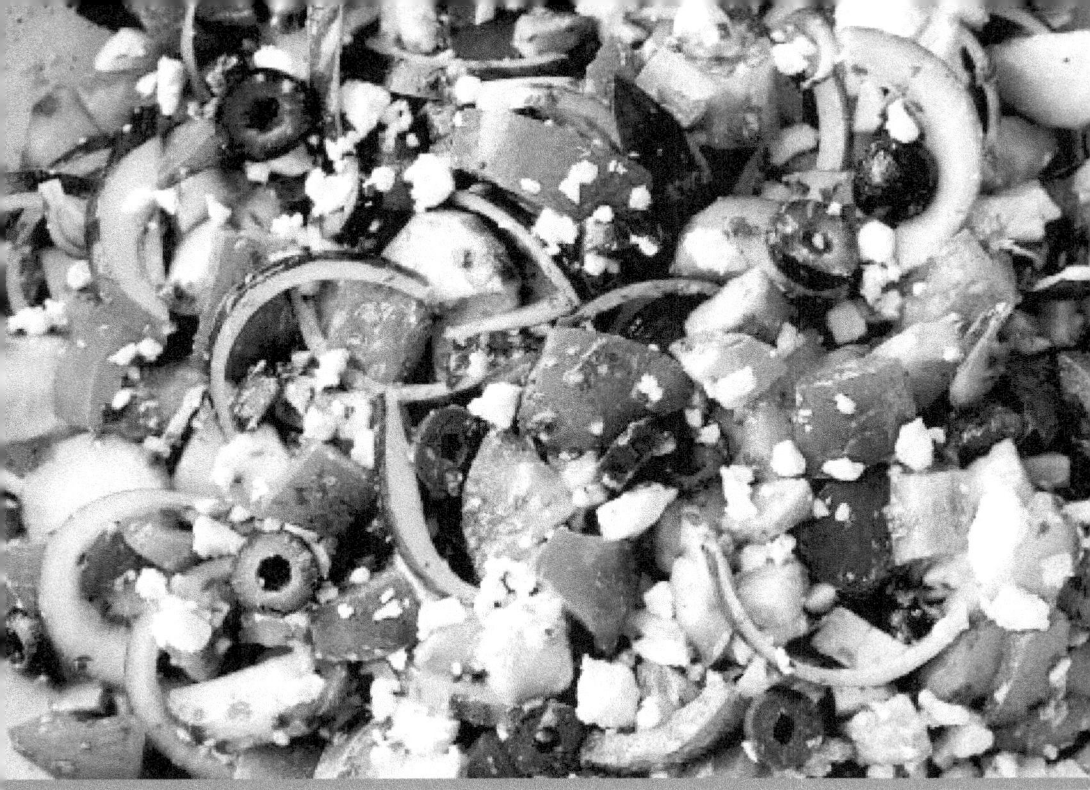

10. GREEK BLACK OLIVE SALAD

Preparation Time: 20 Minutes

Cooking Time: 0 Minutes

Servings: 2

INGREDIENTS:

For the dressing

- 2 tablespoons extra-virgin olive oil
- Juice of 1 lemon
- 1 garlic clove, minced
- 1 teaspoon dried oregano
- Himalayan pink salt
- Freshly ground black pepper

For the salad

- ➢ 1 (15-ounce) can chickpeas, rinsed and drained
- ➢ ⅓ cup pitted kalamata olives or black olives, chopped
- ➢ 1 yellow bell pepper, rinsed and chopped
- ➢ 1 red bell pepper, rinsed and chopped
- ➢ ¼ cup rinsed and diced red onion
- ➢ 15 cherry tomatoes, rinsed, halved, and seeded
- ➢ 1 medium cucumber, rinsed and diced
- ➢ Himalayan pink salt
- ➢ Freshly ground black pepper

DIRECTIONS:

To make the dressing

1. In a small bowl, whisk the olive oil, lemon juice, garlic, and oregano. Season with salt and pepper. Set aside.

To make the salad

2. In a large bowl, stir together the chickpeas, olives, yellow and red bell peppers, red onion, tomatoes, and cucumber.
3. Pour the dressing over the salad and stir again to combine well. Taste and season with salt and pepper. Refrigerate for 1 hour to chill or serve immediately. This salad should last three to five days, covered, in the refrigerator.

NUTRITION:

Calories: 580

Total Fat: 16g

Total Carbohydrates: 93g

Fiber: 27g

Sugar: 28g

Protein: 27g

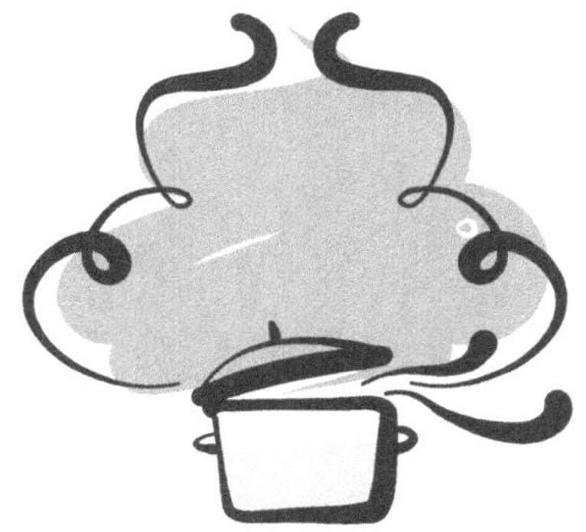

VEGAN CENTRIFUGATES

1. HEARTY ALKALINE STRAWBERRY SUMMER DELUXE

Preparation Time: 5 Minutes

Cooking Time: 20 Minutes

Servings: 2

INGREDIENTS:

- ½ cup organic strawberries/blueberries
- Half of a banana
- 2 cups coconut water
- ½ inch ginger
- Juice of 2 grapefruits

DIRECTIONS:

1. Add all the listed ingredients to your blender
2. Blend until smooth
3. Add a few ice cubes and serve the smoothie
4. Enjoy!

NUTRITION:

Calories 214

Total Fat 10.1 g

Saturated Fat 1.5 g

Cholesterol 0 mg

Sodium 572 mg

Total Carbs 25.3 g

Fiber 4.9 g

Sugar 2.6 g

Protein 4.8 g

2. DELISH PINEAPPLE AND COCONUT MILK SMOOTHIE

Preparation Time: 5 Minutes

Cooking Time: 20 Minutes

Servings: 2

INGREDIENTS:

- ¼ cup pineapple, frozen
- ¾ cup coconut milk

DIRECTIONS:

1. Add the listed ingredients to your blender and blend well with settings on high
2. Once the mixture is smooth, pour the smoothie into a tall glass and serve
3. Chill and enjoy!

NUTRITION:

Calories 274
Total Fat 10.1 g
Saturated Fat 1.5 g
Cholesterol 0 mg
Sodium 572 mg
Total Carbs 25.3 g
Fiber 4.9 g
Sugar 2.6 g
Protein 4.8 g

3. THE MINTY REFRESHER

Preparation Time: 5 Minutes

Cooking Time: 20 Minutes

Servings: 2

INGREDIENTS:

- 2 cups mint tea
- 1 cucumber, peeled
- 2 green apples
- 1 cup blueberries
- Stevia (to sweeten)
- Few slices of lime/lemon for garnish

DIRECTIONS:

1. Add the listed ingredients to your blender and blend until smooth
2. Add ice and sweeten with a bit of stevia
3. Garnish with lime/lemon slices
4. Serve and enjoy!

NUTRITION:

Calories 412

Total Fat 14.1 g

Saturated Fat 1.5 g

Cholesterol 0 mg

Sodium 572 mg

Total Carbs 25.3 g

Fiber 4.9 g

Sugar 2.6 g

Protein 4.8 g

4. THE "UPBEAT" STRAWBERRY AND CLEMENTINE GLASS

Preparation Time: 5 Minutes

Cooking Time: 20 Minutes

Servings: 2

INGREDIENTS:

- 8 ounces strawberries, fresh
- 1 banana, chopped into chunks
- 2 Clementine / Mandarins

DIRECTIONS:

1. Peel the Clementine and remove seeds
2. Add the listed ingredients to your blender/food processor and blend until smooth
3. Serve chilled and enjoy!

NUTRITION:

Calories 344

Total Fat 110.1 g

Saturated Fat 19.5 g

Cholesterol 0 mg

Sodium 572 mg

Total Carbs 25.3 g

Fiber 4.9 g

Sugar 2.6 g

Protein 4.8 g

5. CABBAGE AND COCONUT CHIA SMOOTHIE

Preparation Time: 5 Minutes

Cooking Time: 20 Minutes

Servings: 2

INGREDIENTS:

- 1/3 cup cabbage
- 1 cup cold unsweetened coconut milk
- 1 tablespoon chia seeds
- ½ cup cherries
- ½ cup spinach

DIRECTIONS:

1. Add coconut milk to your blender
2. Cut cabbage and add to your blender
3. Place chia seeds in a coffee grinder and chop to powder, brush the powder into your blender
4. Pit the cherries and add them to your blender
5. Wash and dry the spinach and chop
6. Add to the mix
7. Cover and blend on low followed by medium
8. Taste the texture and serve chilled!

NUTRITION:

Calories 274	Cholesterol 0 mg	Fiber 4.9 g
Total Fat 34.1 g	Sodium 572 mg	Sugar 2.6 g
Saturated Fat 1.5 g	Total Carbs 25.3 g	Protein 4.8 g

6.   THE CHERRY BEET DELIGHT

Preparation Time: 5 Minutes

Cooking Time: 20 Minutes

Servings: 2

INGREDIENTS:

- 1 cup cherries, pitted
- ½ cup beets
- Few bananas slice
- 1 cup water, filtered, alkaline
- 1 cup coconut milk
- Pinch of organic vanilla powder
- Pinch of cinnamon
- Pinch of stevia
- Few mint leaves/lime slices to garnish

DIRECTIONS:

1. Add berries, beets, water, banana slices, coconut milk to your blender
2. Blend well until smooth
3. Add more water if the texture is too creamy for you
4. Add coconut oil, vanilla, cinnamon, and stir
5. Add a bit of stevia for extra sweetness
6. Garnish with mint leaves and lime slices
7. Enjoy!

NUTRITION:

Calories 204	Cholesterol 0 mg	Fiber 4.9 g
Total Fat 10.1 g	Sodium 572 mg	Sugar 2.6 g
Saturated Fat 1.5 g	Total Carbs 25.3 g	Protein 4.8 g

7.   THE AVOCADO PARADISE

Preparation Time: 5 Minutes

Cooking Time: 20 Minutes

Servings: 2

INGREDIENTS:

- ½ avocado, cubed
- 1 cup coconut milk
- Half a lemon
- ¼ cup fresh spinach leaves
- 1 pear
- 1 tablespoon hemp. Seed powder

Toppings

- Handful of macadamia nuts
- Handful of grapes
- 2 lemon slices

DIRECTIONS:

1. Blend all the ingredients until smooth
2. Add a few ice cubes to make it chilled
3. Add your desired toppings
4. Enjoy!

NUTRITION:

Calories 294	Cholesterol 0 mg	Fiber 4.9 g
Total Fat 310.1 g	Sodium 572 mg	Sugar 2.6 g
Saturated Fat 16.5 g	Total Carbs 25.3 g	Protein 4.8 g

8.   THE AUTHENTIC VEGETABLE MEDLEY

Preparation Time: 5 Minutes

Cooking Time: 20 Minutes

Servings: 2

INGREDIENTS:

- 1 cup broccoli, steamed
- 1 bunch asparagus, steamed
- 2 cups coconut milk
- 2 tablespoons coconut oil
- 2 carrots, peeled
- Few inches horseradish
- Himalayan salt
- Pinch of chili powder
- ½ an onion
- 2 garlic cloves

DIRECTIONS:

1. Add all the listed ingredients to your blender except coconut oil, salt and chili powder
2. Blend until smooth
3. Add salt, coconut oil, and chili powder
4. Stir well, and serve chilled!

NUTRITION:

Calories 204

Total Fat 10.1 g

Saturated Fat 1.5 g

Cholesterol 0 mg

Sodium 572 mg

Total Carbs 25.3 g

Fiber 4.9 g

Sugar 2.6 g

Protein 4.8 g

9. THE ORIGINAL POWER PRODUCER

Preparation Time: 5 Minutes

Cooking Time: 20 Minutes

Servings: 2

INGREDIENTS:

- ½ cup spinach
- 1 avocado, diced
- 1 cup coconut milk
- 1 tablespoon flax seed
- 2 nori sheets, roasted and crushed
- 1 garlic clove
- Salt to taste

Toppings

- Handful of pistachios
- 3 tablespoons bell pepper, finely chopped
- A handful of parsley leaves

DIRECTIONS:

1. Blend all the ingredients until smooth
2. Add a few ice cubes to make it chilled
3. Add your desired toppings
4. Enjoy!

NUTRITION:

Calories 224

Total Fat 560.1 g

Saturated Fat 1.5 g

Cholesterol 0 mg

Sodium 572 mg

Total Carbs 25.3 g

Fiber 4.9 g

Sugar 2.6 g

Protein 4.8 g

10. THE DREAMY CHERRY MIX

Preparation Time: 5 Minutes

Cooking Time: 20 Minutes

Servings: 2

INGREDIENTS:

- ½ cup ripe cherries
- Juice of 1 lemon
- 1 cup coconut milk
- 1 avocado, cubed
- ¼ cup spinach
- Few slices of cucumber, peeled

Toppings

- Handful of pistachios
- Handful of raisins
- 1 slice lemon

DIRECTIONS:

1. Blend all the ingredients until smooth
2. Add a few ice cubes to make it chilled
3. Add your desired toppings
4. Enjoy!

NUTRITION:

Calories 232	Cholesterol 0 mg	Fiber 4.9 g
Total Fat 21.1 g	Sodium 572 mg	Sugar 2.6 g
Saturated Fat 16.5 g	Total Carbs 25.3 g	Protein 4.8 g

11. BETTER THAN YOUR FAVORITE RESTAURANT "LEMON SMOOTHIE"

Preparation Time: 5 Minutes

Cooking Time: 20 Minutes

Servings: 2

INGREDIENTS:

- 2 cups organic rice milk, gluten-free
- 1 cup melon, chopped
- ½ an avocado, cubed
- ½ a cucumber, peeled and sliced
- Ice cubes
- 2 limes, juiced
- 1 tablespoon coconut oil
- Few banana slices to taste

DIRECTIONS:

1. Add the listed ingredients to your blender (except coconut oil) and blend well
2. Blend until you have a smooth texture
3. Add coconut oil and stir
4. Enjoy!

NUTRITION:

Calories 204	Cholesterol 0 mg	Fiber 4.9 g
Total Fat 10.1 g	Sodium 572 mg	Sugar 2.6 g
Saturated Fat 1.5 g	Total Carbs 25.3 g	Protein 4.8 g

12. THE "ONE" WITH THE WATERMELON

Preparation Time: 5 Minutes

Cooking Time: 20 Minutes

Servings: 2

INGREDIENTS:

- 1 cup watermelon, sliced
- ½ cup coconut, shredded
- 1 grapefruit, cubed
- ½ cup coconut milk
- 2 tablespoons almond butter

Toppings

- Handful of crushed almonds
- Handful of raisins
- 2 tablespoons coconut powder

DIRECTIONS:

1. Blend all the ingredients until smooth
2. Add a few ice cubes to make it chilled
3. Add your desired toppings
4. Enjoy!

NUTRITION:

Calories 284

Cholesterol 0 mg

Fiber 564.9 g

Total Fat 10.1 g

Sodium 572 mg

Sugar 67.6 g

Saturated Fat 1.5 g

Total Carbs 25.3 g

Protein 14.8 g

13. THE SWEET POTATO ACID BUSTER

Preparation Time: 5 Minutes

Cooking Time: 20 Minutes

Servings: 2

INGREDIENTS:

- 1 cup sweet potato, chopped
- 1 cup almond milk
- ¼ teaspoon nutmeg
- ¼ teaspoon ground cinnamon
- 1 teaspoon flax seed
- 1 small avocado, cubed
- Few spinach leaves, torn
- Toppings
- Handful of crushed almonds
- Handful of crushed cashews
- 3 tablespoons orange juice

DIRECTIONS:

1. Blend all the ingredients until smooth
2. Add a few ice cubes to make it chilled
3. Add your desired toppings
4. Enjoy!

NUTRITION:

Calories 784

Total Fat 10.1 g

Saturated Fat 1.5 g

Cholesterol 0 mg

Sodium 572 mg

Total Carbs 25.3 g

Fiber 564.9 g

Sugar 67.6 g

Protein 14.8 g

14. THE SUNSHINE OFFERING

Preparation Time: 5 Minutes

Cooking Time: 20 Minutes

Servings: 2

INGREDIENTS:

- 2 cups fresh spinach
- 1 and ½ cups almond milk
- ½ cup coconut water
- 3 cups fresh pineapple
- 2 tablespoons coconut unsweetened flakes

DIRECTIONS:

1. Add all the listed ingredients to your blender
2. Blend until smooth
3. Add a few ice cubes and serve the smoothie
4. Enjoy!

NUTRITION:

Calories 784

Total Fat 10.1 g

Saturated Fat 1.5 g

Cholesterol 0 mg

Sodium 572 mg

Total Carbs 25.3 g

Fiber 564.9 g

Sugar 67.6 g

Protein3214.8 g

15. THE SLEEPY BUG SMOOTHIE

Preparation Time: 5 Minutes

Cooking Time: 20 Minutes

Servings: 2

INGREDIENTS:

- 1 cup fennel tea infusion
- 1 cup almond milk
- 1 cup watermelon, chopped
- 1 green apple
- ½ cup pomegranate
- ½ inch ginger
- Stevia to sweeten

DIRECTIONS:

1. Add the listed ingredients to your blender
2. Blend until smooth
3. Add a bit of stevia if you want more sweetness
4. Serve chilled and enjoy!

NUTRITION:

Calories 284

Total Fat 10.1 g

Saturated Fat 1.5 g

Cholesterol 0 mg

Sodium 572 mg

Total Carbs 25.3 g

Fiber 564.9 g

Sugar 67.6 g

Protein 14.8 g

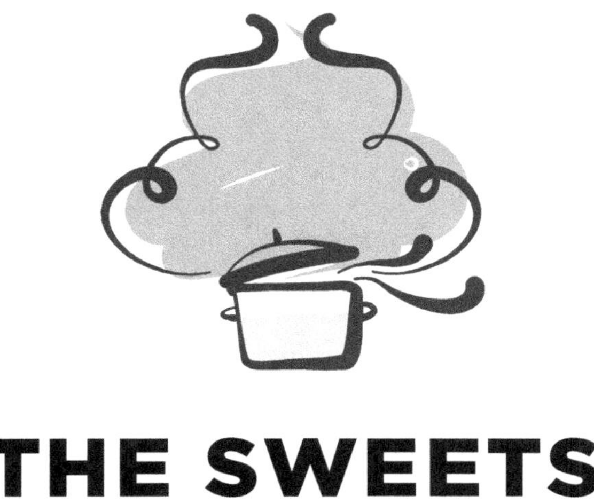

THE SWEETS

1.   STRAWBERRY SORBET

Preparation Time: 4Hours

Cooking Time: 0 Minutes

Servings: 4

INGREDIENTS:

- ➢ 2 cups of Strawberries
- ➢ 1 1/2 teaspoons of Spelt Flour
- ➢ 1/2 cup of Date Sugar
- ➢ 2 cups of Spring Water

DIRECTIONS:

1. Add Date Sugar, Spring Water, and Spelt Flour to a medium pot and boil on low heat for about ten minutes. The mixture should thicken, like syrup.
2. Remove the pot from the heat and allow it to cool.
3. After cooling, add pureed Strawberry and mix gently.
4. Put this mixture in a container and freeze.
5. Cut it into pieces, put the sorbet into a processor and blend until smooth.
6. Put everything back in the container and leave it in the refrigerator for at least four hours.
7. Serve and enjoy your Strawberry Sorbet!

NUTRITION:

Calories: 238

Total Fat: 21g

Total Carbohydrates: 15g

Fiber: 6g

Sugar: 6g

Protein: 2g

2. BLUEBERRY MUFFINS

Preparation Time: 15 Minutes

Cooking Time: 45 Minutes

Servings: 3

INGREDIENTS:

- 1/2 cup of Blueberries
- 3/4 cup of Teff Flour
- 3/4 cup of Spelt Flour
- 1/3 cup of Agave Syrup
- 1/2 teaspoon of Pure Sea Salt
- 1 cup of Coconut Milk
- 1/4 cup of Sea Moss Gel
- Grape Seed Oil

DIRECTIONS:

1. Preheat your oven to 365 degrees Fahrenheit.
2. Grease or line 6 standard muffin cups.
3. Add Teff, Spelt flour, Pure Sea Salt, Coconut Milk, Sea Moss Gel, and Agave Syrup to a large bowl. Mix them together.
4. Add Blueberries to the mixture and mix well.
5. Divide muffin batter among the 6 muffin cups.
6. Bake for 30 minutes until golden brown.
7. Serve and enjoy your Blueberry Muffins!

NUTRITION:

Calories: 600

Total Fat: 45g

Total Carbohydrates: 19g

Fiber: 9g

Sugar: 7g

Protein: 10g

3. BANANA STRAWBERRY ICE CREAM

Preparation Time: 4 Hours

Cooking Time: 0 Minutes

Servings: 5

INGREDIENTS:

- 1 cup of Strawberry
- 5 quartered Baby Bananas
- 1/2 Avocado, chopped
- 1 tablespoon of Agave Syrup
- 1/4 cup of Homemade Walnut Milk

DIRECTIONS:

1. Put all ingredients into the blender and blend them well.
2. Taste. If it is too thick, add extra Milk or Agave Syrup if you want it sweeter.
3. Place in a container with a lid and allow to freeze for at least 5 to 6 hours.
4. Serve it and enjoy your Banana Strawberry Ice Cream!

NUTRITION:

Calories: 470

Total Fat: 17g

Total Carbohydrates: 85g

Fiber: 16g

Sugar: 58g

Protein: 4g

4. HOMEMADE WHIPPED CREAM

Preparation Time: 0 Minutes

Cooking Time: 10 Minutes

Servings: 1 Cup

INGREDIENTS:

- ➢ 1 cup of Aquafaba
- ➢ 1/4 cup of Agave Syrup

DIRECTIONS:

1. Add Agave Syrup and Aquafaba into a bowl.
2. Mix at high speed around 5 minutes with a stand mixer or 10 to 15 minutes with a hand mixer.
3. Serve and enjoy your Homemade Whipped Cream!

NUTRITION:

Calories: 470
Total Fat: 17g
Total Carbohydrates: 85g
Fiber: 16g
Sugar: 58g
Protein: 4g

5. "CHOCOLATE" PUDDING

Preparation Time: 5 Minutes

Cooking Time: 20 Minutes

Servings: 4

INGREDIENTS:

- 1 to 2 cups of Black Sapote
- 1/4 cup of Agave Syrup
- 1/2 cup of soaked Brazil Nuts (overnight or for at least 3 hours)
- 1 tablespoon of Hemp Seeds
- 1/2 cup of Spring Water

DIRECTIONS:

1. Cut 1 to 2 cups of Black Sapote in half.
2. Remove all seeds. You should have 1 full cup of de-seeded fruit.
3. Put all ingredients into a blender and blend until smooth.
4. Serve and enjoy your "Chocolate" Pudding!

NUTRITION:

Calories: 560

Total Fat: 48g

Total Carbohydrates: 31g

Fiber: 22g

Sugar: 5g

Protein: 12g

6. BANANA NUT MUFFINS

Preparation Time: 15 Minutes

Cooking Time: 45 Minutes

Servings: 6

INGREDIENTS:

Dry ingredients:

- 1 1/2 cups of Spell or Teff Flour
- 1/2 teaspoon of Pure Sea Salt
- 3/4 cup of Date Syrup

Wet ingredients:

- 2 medium pureed Burro Bananas
- ¼ cup of Grape Seed Oil
- ¾ *cup of* Homemade Walnut Milk
- 1 tablespoon of Key Lime Juice

Filling ingredients:

- ½ cup of chopped Walnuts (plus extra for decorating)
- 1 chopped Burro Banana

DIRECTIONS:

1. Preheat your oven to 400 degrees Fahrenheit.
2. Take a muffin tray and grease 12 cups or line with cupcake liners.
3. Put all dry ingredients in a large bowl and mix them thoroughly.

4. Add all wet ingredients to a separate, smaller bowl and mix well with pureed Bananas.
5. Mix ingredients from the two bowls in one large container. Be careful not to over mix.
6. Add the filling ingredients and fold in gently.
7. Pour muffin batter into the 12 prepared muffin cups and garnish with a couple of Walnuts.
8. Bake for 22 to 26 minutes until golden brown.
9. Allow to cool for 10 minutes.
10. Serve and enjoy your Banana Nut Muffins!

NUTRITION:

Calories: 470
Total Fat: 17g
Total Carbohydrates: 85g
Fiber: 16g
Sugar: 58g
Protein: 4g

7. MANGO NUT CHEESECAKE

Preparation Time: 30 Minutes

Cooking Time: 4 Hours

Servings: 8

INGREDIENTS:

Filling:

- 2 cups of Brazil Nuts
- 5 to 6 Dates
- 1 tablespoon of Sea Moss Gel
- 1/4 cup of Agave Syrup
- 1/4 teaspoon of Pure Sea Salt
- 2 tablespoons of Lime Juice
- 1 1/2 cups of Homemade Walnut Milk

Crust:

- 1 1/2 cups of quartered Dates
- 1/4 cup of Agave Syrup
- 1 1/2 cups of Coconut Flakes
- 1/4 teaspoon of Pure Sea Salt

Toppings:

- Sliced Mango
- Sliced Strawberries

DIRECTIONS:

1. Put all crust ingredients in a food processor and blend for 30 seconds.
2. Cover a baking form with parchment paper and spread out the blended crust ingredients.
3. Put sliced Mango across the crust and freeze for 10 minutes.
4. Blend all filling ingredients in a blender until smooth.
5. Pour the filling over the crust, cover with foil or parchment paper and let it stand for 3 to 4 hours in the refrigerator.
6. Take out from the baking form and garnish with toppings.
7. Serve and enjoy your Mango Nut Cheesecake!

NUTRITION:

Calories: 650
Total Fat: 48g
Total Carbohydrates: 44g
Fiber: 10g
Sugar: 21g
Protein: 9g

8. BLACKBERRY JAM

Preparation Time: 30 Minutes

Cooking Time: 4 Hours

Servings: 1 Cup

INGREDIENTS:

- ➢ 3/4 cup of Blackberries
- ➢ 1 tablespoon of Key Lime Juice
- ➢ 3 tablespoons of Agave Syrup
- ➢ ¼ cup of Sea Moss Gel + extra 2 tablespoons

DIRECTIONS:

1. Put rinsed Blackberries into a medium pot and cook on medium heat.
2. Stir Blackberries until liquid appears.
3. Once berries soften, use your immersion blender to chop up any large pieces. If you don't have a blender put the mixture in a food processor, mix it well, and then return to the pot.
4. Add Sea Moss Gel, Key Lime Juice, and Agave Syrup to the blended mixture. Boil on medium heat and stir well until it becomes thick.
5. Remove from the heat and leave it to cool for 10 minutes.
6. Serve it with bread pieces or the Flatbread.
7. Enjoy your Blackberry Jam!

NUTRITION:

Calories: 65

Total Fat: 0g

Total Carbohydrates: 16g

Fiber: 3g

Sugar: 12g

Protein: 1g

9. BLACKBERRY BARS

Preparation Time: 20 Minutes

Cooking Time: 60 Minutes

Servings: 4

INGREDIENTS:

- 3 Burro Bananas or 4 Baby Bananas
- 1 cup of Spelt Flour
- 2 cups of Quinoa Flakes
- 1/4 cup of Agave Syrup
- 1/4 teaspoon of Pure Sea Salt
- 1/2 cup of Grape Seed Oil
- 1 cup of prepared Blackberry Jam

DIRECTIONS:

1. Preheat your oven to 350 degrees Fahrenheit.
2. Peel the bananas and mash with a fork in a large bowl.
3. Combine Agave Syrup and Grape Seed Oil with the puree and mix well.
4. Add Spelt Flour and Quinoa Flakes. Knead the dough until it becomes sticky to your fingers.
5. Cover a 9x9-inch baking pan with parchment paper.
6. Take 2/3 of the dough and smooth it out over the parchment pan with your fingers.
7. Spread Blackberry Jam over the dough.
8. Crumble the remaining dough and sprinkle on the top.
9. Bake for 20 minutes.

10. Remove from the oven and let it cool for 10 to 15 minutes.
11. Cut into small pieces.
12. Serve and enjoy your Blackberry Bars!

NUTRITION:

Calories: 98
Total Fat: 4g
Total Carbohydrates: 11g
Fiber: 3g
Sugar: 9g
Protein: 6g

10. SQUASH PIE

Preparation Time: 30 Minutes

Cooking Time: 2 Hours

Servings: 6 to 8

INGREDIENTS:

- 2 Butternut Squashes
- 1 1/4 cups of Spelt Flour
- 1/4 cup of Date Sugar
- 1/4 cup of Agave Syrup
- 1 teaspoon of Allspice
- 1 teaspoon of Pure Sea Salt
- 1/4 cup of Spring Water
- 1/3 cup of Grape Seed Oil
- 1/4 cup of Homemade Hempseed Milk

DIRECTIONS:

Filling:

1. Rinse and peel the Butternut Squashes.
2. Cut them in half and use a spoon to de-seed.
3. Chop the squash into small chunks and add them into a medium pot.
4. Cover the squash in Spring Water and boil it for 20 to 25 minutes until cooked.
5. Pour out the water and mash the cooked squash.
6. Add Date Sugar, Agave Syrup, 1/8 teaspoon of Pure Sea Salt, and Homemade Hempseed Milk and mix them thoroughly.

Crust:

7. Preheat your oven to 350 degrees Fahrenheit.
8. In a bowl, add Spelt Flour, 1/2 teaspoon of Pure Sea Salt, Spring Water, and Grape Seed Oil and mix.
9. Knead dough into a ball. Add more water or flour as needed. Allow it to rest for 5 minutes.
10. Spread out Spelt Flour on a piece of parchment paper.
11. Roll out the dough on the paper by rolling pin, adding more flour to avoid sticking.
12. Place the dough into a pie plate and bake it in the oven for 10 minutes.
13. Remove the crust from the oven, add the pie filling, and bake for another 40 minutes.
14. Remove the pie and leave it for 30 minutes until cool.
15. Serve and enjoy your Squash Pie!

NUTRITION:

Calories: 270
Total Fat: 20g
Total Carbohydrates: 18g
Fiber: 6g
Sugar: 10g
Protein: 5g

CONCLUSION

Often, we tend to neglect our health and only realize that we have to make important changes when it's already too late. Whenever we go about our regular day-to-day activities, we think about what we need to do and the things we have to accomplish next, without even giving a single thought to how we are treating our bodies. But when our systems start to fail, and our bodies start to break down, only then do we see just how important it is to take care of ourselves from seemingly insignificant details like the hours of sleep we take to the kind of food we ingest.

We slave day after day to work and toil, and when we fall ill, all we do is try to find ways to get better with expensive medicines and complicated chemicals. The best thing to do is to prevent these ailments altogether using all-natural means to stay healthy—after all, why should we make our bodies take in even more chemicals in order to get rid of the chemicals that are already there?

Further, chemicals like artificial sweeteners and flavorings, food colorings, preservatives, and other substances inflame the body, toxify the liver, and leave us vulnerable to a long list of diseases. If you love eating nutrient-dense foods, the alkaline diet is a great diet for you.

If you want to know just how healthy the alkaline diet could be for you, consider how long people live in areas of the world called "the Blue Zones." These five areas—the Ogliastra region of Sardinia; Ikaria,

Greece; Okinawa, Japan; Nicoya Peninsula, Costa Rica; and Loma Linda, California—boast the longest-living people in the world. And all share one thing in common: a diet chiefly of alkalizing vegetables.

The alkaline diet has proven to be life-altering for the better. I found that eating an alkaline, plant-based diet was a great way to experience easy weight loss and maintain a slim body, high energy, clear skin, and complete vitality. I have had a new enthusiasm for life, exercise, goals, hobbies, and relationships since I started on an alkaline diet almost two decades ago.

I would like to thank you for purchasing the book and taking the time for going through it as well. I do hope that this book has been helpful and you found the information contained in the recipes useful! Keep in mind that you are not only limited to the recipes provided in this book!

It's also helped my mood, be more positive and stable, and I've seen a newfound sense of general "happiness for no reason" on this diet as well. I've designed this text for the person who wants to try the alkaline life but wants an easy guide that takes them step-by-step through the process of what to eat, how to eat, and how to test your alkalinity/ acidity to see if you're on track. I wish you all my best and welcome to a high-energy way to live lighter (and longer) on your feet.

www.ingramcontent.com/pod-product-compliance
Lightning Source LLC
Chambersburg PA
CBHW061804250726
48657CB00001B/273